D1592666

INTEGRATED GROUP THERAPY
FOR BIPOLAR DISORDER AND SUBSTANCE ABUSE

'SCARD

DISCARD

Integrated Group Therapy for Bipolar Disorder and Substance Abuse

ROGER D. WEISS

HILARY SMITH CONNERY

THE GUILFORD PRESS

New York   London

PROPERTY OF WLU
SOCIAL WORK LIBRARY

DISCARD

© 2011 The Guilford Press
A Division of Guilford Publications, Inc.
72 Spring Street, New York, NY 10012
www.guilford.com

All rights reserved

Except as indicated, no part of this book may be reproduced, translated, stored in a retrieval
system, or transmitted, in any form or by any means, electronic, mechanical, photocopying,
microfilming, recording, or otherwise, without written permission from the publisher.

Printed in the United States of America

This book is printed on acid-free paper.

Last digit is print number: 9 8 7 6 5 4 3 2 1

LIMITED PHOTOCOPY LICENSE

These materials are intended for use only by qualified professionals.

The publisher grants to individual purchasers of this book nonassignable permission to
reproduce all materials for which photocopying permission is specifically granted in a
footnote. This license is limited to you, the individual purchaser, for personal use or use
with individual clients or students. This license does not grant the right to reproduce these
materials for resale, redistribution, electronic display, or any other purposes (including
but not limited to books, pamphlets, articles, video- or audiotapes, bogs, file-sharing sites,
Internet or intranet sites, and handouts or slides for lectures, workshops, webinars, or
therapy groups, whether or not a fee is charged). Permission to reproduce these materials for
these and any other purposes must be obtained in writing from the Permissions Department
of Guilford Publications.

The authors have checked with sources believed to be reliable in their efforts to provide
information that is complete and generally in accord with the standards of practice that are
accepted at the time of publication. However, in view of the possibility of human error or
changes in behavioral, mental health, or medical sciences, neither the authors, nor the editor and
publisher, nor any other party who has been involved in the preparation or publication of this
work warrants that the information contained herein is in every respect accurate or complete, and
they are not responsible for any errors or omissions or the results obtained from the use of such
information. Readers are encouraged to confirm the information contained in this book with other
sources.

Library of Congress Cataloging-in-Publication Data

Weiss, Roger D., 1951– author.
    Integrated group therapy for bipolar disorder and substance abuse / Roger D. Weiss,
Hilary Smith Connery.
        p. ; cm.
    Includes bibliographical references and index.
    ISBN 978-1-60918-060-7 (pbk.: alk. paper)
    1. Manic–depressive illness—Treatment.   2. Substance abuse—Treatment.   3. Group
psychotherapy.   I. Connery, Hilary Smith, author.   II. Title.
    [DNLM: 1. Bipolar Disorder—therapy.   2. Psychotherapy, Group—methods.
3. Substance-Related Disorders—therapy.   WM 207]
    RC516.W39 2011
    616.89′506—dc22

                                                                  2010047291

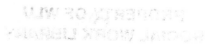

To Barb and Les, Em and Al, and Maggie, with love

To Barb and Ger, great mentors of perseverance

About the Authors

Roger D. Weiss, MD, is Professor of Psychiatry at Harvard Medical School and Chief of the Division of Alcohol and Drug Abuse at McLean Hospital in Belmont, Massachusetts. Through his research, international teaching, clinical work, and writings, Dr. Weiss has made significant contributions to the field of substance use disorders, with a particular focus on those individuals with co-occurring psychiatric illness. He has been Principal Investigator on numerous National Institute on Drug Abuse and National Institute on Alcohol Abuse and Alcoholism grants, and he recently led a multisite national study of the treatment of prescription opioid dependence as part of the National Institute on Drug Abuse Clinical Trials Network. He has authored over 300 articles and book chapters and has participated in a number of prominent national committees, including serving as vice chair of the American Psychiatric Association Task Force on Practice Guidelines for Patients with Substance Use Disorders. In 2007, the Centre for Addiction and Mental Health in Toronto selected Dr. Weiss as the recipient of the H. David Archibald Award for Outstanding Research and/or Practice in the Addictions.

Hilary Smith Connery, MD, PhD, is Clinical Director of the Alcohol and Drug Abuse Treatment Program at McLean Hospital in Belmont, Massachusetts, and Instructor in Psychiatry at Harvard Medical School. Dr. Connery is a clinical researcher who studies innovative behavioral treatments for patients with co-occurring substance use disorders and mental illness. She has special interest in the treatment of patients with opioid dependence and mental illness and has been a recipient of the Eleanor and Miles Shore/Harvard Medical Scholars Fellowship to study this population. She participated as site Principal Investigator on two national studies of buprenorphine treatment of opioid dependence through the National Institute on Drug Abuse Clinical Trials Network, and she is co-investigator on other federally funded clinical research studies addressing substance use treatment in women and medically ill individuals. Dr. Connery also has community psychiatry experience running assertive community treatment teams and studying barriers to recovery among homeless persons. She is currently listed in Best Doctors in America, is a consultant to the Massachusetts Board of Registration in Medicine and the National Football League, and is Area 1 Director for the American Academy of Addiction Psychiatry.

Preface

This book is designed to teach people how to conduct Integrated Group Therapy (IGT), a 12-session group treatment for individuals with co-occurring bipolar disorder and substance abuse problems. The book begins by presenting an overview of IGT and reviewing basic information about bipolar disorder, substance abuse, and cognitive-behavioral therapy, which is the theoretical model underlying IGT. The second chapter consists of a more detailed discussion of the guiding principles behind IGT and reviews the general conduct of an IGT session.

Following the introductory chapters is a detailed session-by-session guide to conducting each of the 12 IGT group sessions. Included are guidelines about group size, length of sessions, choosing a patient population, responding to substance use by group members, dealing with disruptive patients, and handling emergencies such as suicidal ideation. We then present (and answer) a list of "Frequently Asked Questions" about IGT and offer a guide to help therapists monitor whether they are conducting IGT as intended. Finally, the book closes with reference material and guides for further reading and assistance.

Bipolar disorder is the psychiatric illness associated with the highest risk of co-occurring substance abuse problems. Those with co-occurring bipolar and substance use disorders typically have poorer outcomes—more hospitalizations, more homelessness, and a greater risk of suicide—than those with either disorder alone. Despite the high rate of co-occurrence and the associated negative consequences, very little research had previously been conducted to develop a treatment—either medication or counseling—for this population. This book thus represents an important step to remedy this situation.

Two randomized, controlled trials—the gold standard for clinical research—have shown that IGT has produced better outcomes than standard group drug counseling. Developed at the Alcohol and Drug Abuse Treatment Program at McLean Hospital in Belmont, Massachusetts, a teaching hospital of Harvard Medical School, IGT is now used in multiple treatment programs in the United States and Canada. We are hopeful that as a result of our publication of this book, more treatment programs will have the opportunity to use IGT for this dually diagnosed patient population.

Acknowledgments

This book is a result of over a decade's worth of work, accomplished by dozens of people. We are grateful to Lisa Onken and Jack Blaine at the Behavioral Therapies Development Program of the National Institute on Drug Abuse (NIDA) for their support; NIDA funding (Grant Nos. R01 DA09400, R01 DA15968, K02 DA00326, and K24 DA022288) enabled us to develop Integrated Group Therapy (IGT) and to conduct the studies that established its effectiveness. We are also grateful to the Dr. Ralph and Marian C. Falk Medical Research Trust for their generous support of our early work in the development of IGT.

These studies were successful because of the efforts of a team of investigators, research coordinators, and therapists who carried out the research. Although many people were involved, Shelly Greenfield, the first person to lead an IGT group, and Lisa Najavits, who contributed a great deal to the theoretical vision of IGT, were important collaborators early in the process of developing IGT. John Rodolico, one of the initial IGT therapists, did a superb job training and supervising subsequent therapists in later studies. Dennis Daley from the University of Pittsburgh skillfully trained and supervised group leaders for Group Drug Counseling, our comparison condition for IGT. Monika Kolodziej and Bill Jaffee conducted diagnostic assessments and oversaw much of the evaluation process that was so important in determining the level of success of our intervention. Steve Strakowski and Eduard Vieta, both leaders in bipolar disorder research, provided helpful advice at various stages of the research process. Garrett Fitzmaurice, Bob Gallop, and the late John Hennen all provided invaluable guidance in data analysis.

We were very fortunate to have an extraordinarily talented group of research coordinators throughout the process of developing and studying IGT. This bright, personable, and enthusiastic group of young men and women were responsible for conducting the studies day by day: recruiting patients for the study, interviewing them throughout the study, entering data, scheduling appointments, and responding to emergencies; they provided the glue that kept the studies going. Margaret Griffin directed the studies: training and supervising the research coordinators, keeping the studies on track, ensuring that data collection was carried out properly, analyzing data, and making sure that these studies represented the highest possible quality research.

Finally, we are grateful to the patients who put their faith in us and in the research process by choosing to enter our studies. Clinical research and the development of new treatments cannot proceed without people who volunteer to participate in treatment studies. We thus owe our patients a great deal, and we are pleased that the result of these studies—the establishment of a new effective treatment for those with bipolar disorder and substance abuse problems—will now be available to a much wider population.

Contents

xiv   Contents

INTEGRATED GROUP THERAPY
FOR BIPOLAR DISORDER AND SUBSTANCE ABUSE

PART I

OVERVIEW OF INTEGRATED GROUP THERAPY

CHAPTER 1

⦿⦿⦿⦿⦿⦿⦿⦿⦿⦿⦿⦿⦿⦿⦿⦿

An Introduction to Integrated Group Therapy

This book offers step-by-step guidelines for conducting Integrated Group Therapy (IGT), an evidence-based treatment for patients with co-occurring bipolar disorder (BD) and substance use disorder (SUD). Designed to be delivered by substance abuse counselors as well as other mental health professionals, IGT consists of 12 one-hour group sessions. IGT stresses the importance of dealing with both psychiatric and substance use problems simultaneously, and looks for common themes in the development of these two illnesses as well as in the course of recovery from and relapse to both disorders.

The major goals of IGT are (1) to promote abstinence from drugs of abuse, including alcohol; (2) to promote adherence to medications prescribed for BD; (3) to teach symptom recognition for the purpose of both sustaining mood stability and SUD relapse prevention; (4) to teach skills that facilitate SUD relapse prevention (e.g., drug and alcohol refusal skills, avoidance of high-risk situations) as well as mood stability (e.g., prioritizing protective routines, such as sleep hygiene, over high-risk social behavior); and (5) to improve other aspects of life functioning, including interpersonal relationships. IGT is designed to be administered in conjunction with pharmacological treatment for BD as well as other treatments that a patient may receive, such as individual psychotherapy, other group treatment, and self-help/mutual-help support groups.

IGT fills a need for an effective treatment specifically designed for this population. While there are effective research-based treatments for BD as well as those for SUDs, patients with this comorbidity have posed treatment challenges. IGT has been cited by the National Institute on Drug Abuse (2009) as one of only five examples of "promising behavioral therapies for adult patients with comorbid conditions" (p. 3). It is the only treatment for patients with co-occurring BD and SUDs with a substantial evidence base demonstrating its efficacy, including research showing that it can be successfully implemented by properly trained front-line substance abuse counselors. Patients enjoy IGT, and clinicians like learning it and conducting it. Most importantly, as we detail later in this chapter, patients receiving IGT have been shown to attain better outcomes than have those who received standard group substance abuse counseling.

3

THE PROBLEM OF CO-OCCURRING
BIPOLAR AND SUBSTANCE USE DISORDERS

A number of studies, including surveys of community samples (Grant, Stinson, et al., 2004; Kessler, Crum, et al., 1997) and studies of patients seeking treatment (Cassidy, Ahearn, et al., 2001), have consistently shown that SUDs and BD frequently occur together. In fact, the Epidemiologic Catchment Area study, conducted by the National Institute of Mental Health, revealed that BD was the psychiatric illness most likely to co-occur with an SUD (Regier, Farmer, et al., 1990). In that study, the likelihood of an individual with BD having an SUD was more than six times greater than that of the general population. People with bipolar I disorder (i.e., those who have been hospitalized for mania) had an even higher risk: they were nearly eight times more likely than those in the general population to have an SUD.

What accounts for this? What is it about having a psychiatric illness that predisposes people to having an SUD? Multiple factors may contribute to this phenomenon. One possibility is that BD and SUD carry a common genetic vulnerability; both of these disorders are known to run in families, and a number of studies have pointed to genetic contributions to these disorders. A second contributing factor is the possibility that some people with psychiatric illness may initially find specific substances of abuse to be particularly rewarding. In addition to the usual reinforcing properties of substances of abuse, some people initially find that particular substances temporarily relieve some of their painful psychiatric symptoms. Thus, if someone with BD believes that cocaine temporarily lifts depressed mood, or that marijuana temporarily slows down racing thoughts or reduces irritability, then that person might be more likely to continue taking that drug, even if (as is often the case) the substance later turns out to be both less successful at relieving these symptoms and prone to cause other problems. The use of substances in an attempt to relieve unwanted psychiatric symptoms is frequently referred to as *self-medication*, a term that was popularized by Edward Khantzian at Harvard Medical School in the 1980s (Khantzian, 1985). In our experience, many patients who seek treatment for BD and SUD describe their substance use as an attempt at self-medication.

Although self-medication may successfully relieve psychiatric symptoms at first, drugs of abuse are not effective long-term treatments; they often actually *increase* psychiatric symptoms over time rather than reducing them. This does not always stop people from continuing to use these substances, however. For some individuals who realize that substance-induced mood improvement is no longer possible (because the drugs stop working in this way), mood *change* may become the goal of substance use. Indeed, many patients have described the use of alcohol or drugs during a period of depression as a means of "numbing out," or blotting out feelings rather than experiencing actual mood improvement. As one patient said, "I just don't want to feel anything right now. If I drink enough, I won't have to think about how depressed I am. I know I'll feel worse tomorrow, but I just don't care." This type of statement reveals the sense of hopelessness that many patients feel. Patients with BD and substance dependence often experience what we call "layers of hopelessness" (Weiss, 2004). First, they may feel hopeless about being able to stop using drugs or alcohol. Then they feel hopeless that their lives will improve, even if they actually *do* stop their substance use; they believe that they have dug a deep hole for themselves and cannot escape. Finally, they have the global sense of overarching hopelessness that many patients with depression experience as a symptom of their illness. These layers of hopelessness lead people to believe that they are unable to improve their lives; it therefore does not matter what they do. This dynamic of feeling hopeless and therefore not taking action is one of the central themes that need to be addressed when treating this population.

Finally, patients with psychiatric illness often display poor judgment. This is most obvious during periods of mania, when people may spend large amounts of money that they don't have, and may engage in sexual indiscretions and other forms of risky behavior, including substance use. People with severe anxiety or depression can have poor judgment as well, because they are not thinking clearly about their future and may act on the basis of panic or a sense of hopelessness about the future. They may thus make poor decisions about substances that they would not make when asymptomatic. This phenomenon represents one of the great challenges when treating patients with co-occurring psychiatric illness and SUDs: people may be highly enthusiastic and motivated for abstinence while engaged in treatment, when their psychiatric symptoms may be under good control. However, they may lose their resolve during a psychiatric crisis, when their decision-making capabilities are compromised.

Multiple studies have shown that patients with BD who also abuse alcohol or drugs are at greater risk for poor outcomes. Such individual are more likely to have a slow recovery from mood episodes (Keller, Lavori, et al., 1986), are twice as likely to require hospitalization (Brady, Casto, et al., 1991), and have a higher rate of poor adherence to their medication regimens (Keck, McElroy, et al., 1997); the latter is known to predict poorer outcomes in this population (Keck, McElroy, et al., 1998). Finally, patients with BD and SUD are also at greater risk for suicidal behavior (Dalton, Cate-Carter, et al., 2003). Thus, finding an effective treatment for this population has been a significant public health priority.

What We Know about Treatment of Co-Occurring Bipolar and Substance Use Disorders

Despite the high rate of co-occurrence of BD and SUDs, very little treatment research has specifically targeted this dually diagnosed population. There have only been a handful of medication trials, and most of them were extremely small (20 patients or fewer). Perhaps the best known study of medication for this population was performed by Ihsan Salloum and his colleagues at the University of Pittsburgh (Salloum, Cornelius, et al., 2005). These researchers studied 59 patients with BD and alcohol dependence, all of whom were treated with the mood stabilizer lithium. In addition to lithium, half of the trial participants were randomly assigned to another mood stabilizer, valproate; half received lithium plus a placebo pill. Salloum and his colleagues found that the patients who received lithium plus valproate had fewer days of heavy drinking and a trend toward fewer drinks on their heavy drinking days. This study has commonly been misinterpreted as showing that valproate was better than lithium for this population; this is not what was found, however. Rather, all patients in this particular study received lithium, and it was the addition of valproate that improved drinking outcomes. A more recent study by E. Sherwood Brown and his colleagues at the University of Texas Southwestern Medical School (Brown, Garza, et al., 2008), found that the atypical antipsychotic medication quetiapine was not better than placebo at improving drinking outcomes in patients with BD and alcohol use disorder. However, quetiapine may have been helpful in reducing depressive symptoms in this population.

In the past 20 years, there has been intense interest in psychotherapy and other kinds of behavioral therapies for people with BD; substance dependence has generated similar research interest. However, as with pharmacotherapy, there has been virtually no research on psychosocial treatments specifically designed for patients with both disorders. A number of different types of psychotherapy have been found to be quite helpful as adjunctive treatments to pharmacotherapy for patients with BD. These include group psychoeducation (Colom, Vieta, et al., 2003), family-focused treatment (Miklowitz, Otto, et al., 2007), individual interpersonal and social rhythm therapy (Frank, Kupfer, et al., 2005), and cognitive-behavioral therapy (CBT; Lam, Watkins, et al., 2003). Overall, these psychotherapies for BD have been shown to produce a lower relapse rate, a reduction in mood symptoms, and better social and relational functioning (Lam, Burbeck, et al., 2009). While most of these psychotherapy studies have included patients with SUDs, and all address the harmful role of substance abuse in BD, none focus primarily on that issue.

A number of behavioral therapies for SUDs also have a strong evidence base of success, including motivational enhancement therapy (Dunn, Deroo et al., 2001; Hettema, Steele, et al., 2005), CBT (Dutra, Stathopoulou, et al., 2008), 12-step facilitation (Ferri, Amato, et al., 2006), disease-oriented individual drug counseling (Crits-Christoph, Siqueland, et al., 1999), contingency management (Dutra, Stathopoulou, et al., 2008), and behavioral couples therapy (Powers, Vedel, et al., 2008), among others. Most studies of patients with SUDs either exclude patients with BD or have a very small number of patients with BD, so it is unclear whether these treatments are useful for that subpopulation.

The treatment of patients with SUD and co-occurring psychiatric illness is frequently divided in its delivery (Drake, Mueser, et al., 1996). It may occur sequentially (e.g., the patient receives SUD treatment, followed by treatment for BD) or in parallel (the patient simultaneously receives treatment for each disorder in two different settings). Sequential treatment offers the advantage of attending to the most acute disorder, but the second disorder may not be addressed adequately. Parallel treatment also presents a number of difficulties. For example, mental health treatment programs may minimize the significance of substance use, while substance abuse treatment staff members may overattribute psychiatric symptoms to substance use. A number of clinicians and researchers have thus recommended *integrated treatment* for dually diagnosed patients—that is, treatment of both disorders at the same time in the same setting by the same treater or group of clinicians, who are familiar with both disorders (Brunette & Mueser, 2006). Although this approach has been advocated for nearly 20 years (Mueser, Bellack, et al., 1992), only recently has there been a substantial number of empirical studies of integrated treatment for dually diagnosed patients.

In the rest of this chapter, we provide information on BD, its definition, course, and treatment, followed by similar information on SUDs. We then discuss integrated treatments in general and IGT in particular, including research on its effectiveness. Chapter 2 reviews the nature of IGT, including its theoretical foundation, major themes, and key considerations in conducting the treatment. Chapter 3 reviews the pregroup interview and includes Handout 1, entitled "Ways to Benefit from This Treatment." Chapter 4 is a step-by-step guide to conducting an IGT session. Part II of the book presents detailed guidelines for conducting the 12 IGT sessions and includes copies of patient handouts. This is followed by three Appendices, including a rating form for therapists to assess their performance in IGT (Appendix A), which can be helpful in supervision for performance improvement; bulletin board material (Appendix B), some for use in all IGT sessions and some for specific sessions; and a series of frequently asked questions about IGT (Appendix C).

BIPOLAR DISORDER

BD affects approximately 5.7 million American adults each year (Kessler, Crum, et al., 1997), representing 8.1% of all diagnosed mental illness (U.S. Department of Health and Human Services, 1999) in the United States. Previously called "manic–depression" or "manic–depressive illness," BD can present in a variety of ways, making diagnosis challenging. In this section, we define the disorder and its natural course, and review current theories about its etiology. We also discuss important clinical aspects of BD, such as increased risk of suicide and the high incidence of co-occurring SUDs. Finally, we provide a brief review of current treatments in use for BD.

Defining Bipolar Disorder

The active phases of BD are characterized by abnormalities in mood, thought, emotion, and energy; these abnormalities are recognizable by observable changes in behavior and by self-report. The distinguishing feature of BD is the cyclical course between depressive symptoms (most often manifesting as a slowing in thought and energy, and sad or blunted emotion) and symptoms in the manic phase (often manifesting as racing thoughts, rapid speech, increased energy, and labile emotions). The fourth edition of the American Psychiatric Association's (2000) *Diagnostic and Statistical Manual of Mental Disorders* (DSM-IV-TR) lists four distinct subcategories of BD (bipolar I, bipolar II, cyclothymic disorder, and bipolar disorder not otherwise specified), defined by episodes of depression, mania, hypomania, or mixed symptom episodes. The criteria defining these episodes are reviewed below.

Manic Episode

A *manic episode* involves a period of "elevated, expansive, or irritable" mood lasting at least a week and/or causing enough impairment of functioning as to require hospitalization. Manic symptoms may include grandiosity, reduced need for sleep, racing thoughts, rapid, pressured speech, and engagement in risky activities such as spending sprees or sexual indiscretions. Full criteria for these and other disorders described in this manual can be found in the DSM-IV-TR manual (American Psychiatric Association, 2000).

Hypomanic Episode

A *hypomanic episode* can be difficult to distinguish from a manic episode. The major distinction between the two is severity of symptoms, with hypomania characterized by less severe disruption of functioning than mania. The symptom criteria are the same as those for a manic episode (see preceding subsection), but the period marked by elevated, expansive, or irritable mood may be limited to 4 days in duration. As with a manic episode, the symptoms may not be due to the effects of a substance or a medical condition.

Major Depressive Episode

A major depressive episode consists of a 2-week period in which an individual reports being depressed fairly consistently throughout much of the day; symptoms include changes in appetite or sleep (either an increase or decrease), a lack of energy, a sense of restlessness or agitation, a reduced ability to experience pleasure, and morbid thoughts, which may include suicidal ideas or behavior. A major depressive episode ordinarily interferes with functioning, although the level of severity of dysfunction can be highly variable. In severe cases, people with a major depressive episode may struggle to accomplish basic tasks such as getting out of bed.

Mixed Episode

A *mixed episode* is defined as a 1-week period in which a person meets criteria for both a manic episode *and* a major depressive episode. The symptoms listed earlier for a manic episode and a depressive episode may occur simultaneously; thus, a person may report feeling unusually energetic but also feel worthless. Again, this disturbance must impair a person's usual functional capacities and not be due to substance use or a medical condition.

The course and combination of these episodes determine the particular diagnosis of BD a person receives. If an individual has had at least one manic or mixed episode, he or she qualifies for a bipolar I diagnosis. An individual with this diagnosis usually has also suffered at least one major depressive episode; however, a major depressive episode is not necessary for a diagnosis of BD. An individual who has experienced at least one hypomanic episode, as well as at least one major depressive episode, qualifies for a bipolar II diagnosis; any manic or mixed episode excludes bipolar II disorder in favor of bipolar I disorder.

Cyclothymic disorder is diagnosed when symptoms of hypomania and depression are present, but not in quantity or severity sufficient to meet criteria for a full manic, major depressive, or mixed episode. Additionally, an individual must experience these mood symptoms for at least 2 years, while having no more than 2 consecutive symptom-free months. In some cases, cyclothymic disorder may progress to bipolar I or II disorder over time, as symptom intensity worsens. If someone has met these criteria for the initial 2 years of mood difficulties and subsequently experiences a more serious disturbance (e.g., a manic episode), then that individual would be diagnosed with both cyclothymic disorder and bipolar I disorder.

BD not otherwise specified is the diagnosis used for an individual who has identifiable features of BD but does not meet full criteria for any of the previously described disorders. For example, a person shifting between manic and depressive symptoms over the course of a few days without meeting episode criteria, and having significant periods of symptom remission, does not meet criteria for cyclothymic disorder and would receive a diagnosis of BD not otherwise specified. A person with a history of only hypomanic episodes, and no depression, would likewise receive a diagnosis of BD not otherwise specified. The diagnosis of BD not otherwise specified may have particular relevance for the dually diagnosed population that participates in IGT. For patients in whom it is difficult to determine whether mood symptoms would be clinically significant without their substance use, then BD not otherwise specified could be a "working" or temporary diagnosis while they are observed over time. This strategy can be particularly helpful if they are able to achieve abstinence from drugs and alcohol, since the mood symptoms can then be evaluated both on and off substances.

Since many substances of abuse can cause profound changes in mood, thinking, and behavior, diagnosing BD in the presence of active substance abuse can be challenging. This is particularly true among those who abuse central nervous system stimulants such as cocaine and methamphetamine, which can mimic some of the symptoms of BD. Thus, when taking a history in patients with SUDs, it is important to try to determine the relation between mood symptoms and substance use. To the degree that mood symptoms correlate strongly with substance use patterns that could reasonably be expected to produce these symptoms, then the diagnosis of BD becomes more questionable. For example, in someone whose mood symptoms occur only in the context of cocaine binges, a diagnosis of substance-induced mood disorder would likely be most appropriate. Similarly, mood symptoms that occur only in the context of major shifts in substance use (e.g., increases or decreases in drinking) might represent a substance-induced mood disorder as well. In contrast, if someone has experienced symptoms characteristic of BD in the face of relatively steady use (e.g., a regular pattern of drinking six beers per night), or if the intensity or length of symptoms exceeds what would be expected as a result of an individual's particular substance use pattern, then the diagnosis of BD likely should be made. It is important to note that there are many gray areas here. Patients commonly do not remember clearly the temporal relation between their substance use and mood episodes; you are likely to hear answers such as "I've been depressed for a long time and I've been drinking for a long time, and I can't really remember what leads to what." In such instances, following a patient over time may be the only way to distinguish between substance-induced and independent mood symptoms.

Causes of Bipolar Disorder

Bipolar disorder is heritable; individuals who have a family member with BD are more likely to be diagnosed with BD at some point in their lifetime, and there is increasing evidence for the role of genetic variations that contribute to vulnerability to BD (Craddock, O'Donovan, et al., 2005). Environmental factors also play a role in the etiology of BD. For example, while we know that the identical twin of someone with BD is at greater risk to have BD, many identical twins of those with BD do not have the disorder. If BD were a purely genetic disorder, then all identical twins of those with BD would also have the disorder.

The Course of Bipolar Disorder

BD is a chronic mental illness, and appropriate ongoing treatment with medication is ordinarily required to help a person to function normally. In fact, without medical treatment, the average person with bipolar I disorder will have at least four acute episodes (either manic or major depressive) within 10 years (American Psychiatric Association, 2000), resulting in significant morbidity or mortality. Although medication treatment clearly improves prognosis dramatically, many people with BD continue to have difficulties with functioning despite adequate pharmacotherapy, and relapses can occur despite good pharmacotherapy and high levels of medication adherence (Goldberg & Harrow, 2004).

The average age of onset for BD is 25 years old (Kessler, Crum, et al., 1997), although BD may sometimes be diagnosed during childhood or adolescence; this is frequently associated with irritable mood (Birmaher, Axelson, et al., 2009). BD is equally common among men and women. The term *polarity* is often used to describe the course of illness; *mania* and *depres-*

sion are two opposite poles of one disorder (hence the name *bipolar*). Shifts between the two poles can occur either in sequence (i.e., a "manic switch" directly from a depressed episode, or a "depressive crash" at the end of a manic episode) or after a period of symptom remission between episodes (*euthymia*, or normal good mood). Over the course of the illness, depression typically becomes more predominant. Indeed, dealing with depression is a core theme of IGT, since many patients entering this group have had BD for a substantial period of time and therefore suffer more frequently from depression than from mania.

Suicide Risk

Untreated BD can be highly lethal: a recent, large outpatient community study found suicide completion rates of 0.14% per year for bipolar I disorder and even higher, 0.16% per year, for bipolar II disorder (Tondo, Lepri, et al., 2007). The relative risk for completed suicide in this sample was approximately 15 times greater than that of the general population. Thus, suicidal thoughts and feelings of hopelessness, isolation, and despair must be aggressively assessed and treated when working with patients with BD. It is important to note that suicidal ideation can occur during *any* mood episode and is not limited to depressive episodes.

The risk of suicidal behavior in patients with BD increases with a co-occurring SUD (Neves, Malloy-Diniz, et al., 2009), and an individual with BD is up to eight times more likely than the general population to develop a co-occurring SUD during his or her lifetime (Kessler, Crum, et al., 1997; Regier, Farmer, et al., 1990). Patients with BD are more likely to make a violent suicide attempt (hanging, jumping from a high place, cutting themselves) when there is co-occurring alcohol dependence (Neves, Malloy-Diniz, et al., 2009). Therefore, diagnosing a co-occurring SUD and helping an individual to achieve and maintain abstinence is an important aspect of suicide prevention and mood stabilization.

Treatment

The treatment of BD can be categorized into three phases: psychiatric management, acute treatment, and maintenance treatment.

Psychiatric Management

This phase of treatment comes after diagnosis and involves creating a treatment plan, providing individuals and their families and partners with educational information about BD, and teaching them how to identify symptoms of BD and avoid common triggers of mood episodes.

Acute Treatment

When an individual is experiencing a manic or mixed episode, treatment with medication is the first-line response. Several antimanic medications are effective, including mood stabilizers such as lithium carbonate, valproate, and the antipsychotic class of medications. Sedative–hypnotic benzodiazepines are also commonly used acutely as an adjunct to aid with patient comfort and/ or behavioral control. A single medication or a combination of more than one may be prescribed.

Electroconvulsive therapy (ECT) may also be administered in severe cases or for individuals who do not respond to medications. A similar approach is used for a patient with a depressive episode, although the mood stabilizer lamotrigine has shown evidence of efficacy for bipolar depression (Geddes, Calabrese, et al., 2009). Maintenance of patient safety and suicide precautions are always prescribed, regardless of the type of acute episode.

Maintenance Treatment

Following acute stabilization of an episode, an individual should remain in an ongoing treatment plan that further supports symptom remission. This plan usually includes a regimen of the medications used to treat acute episodes (perhaps combined with ECT), as well as a psychosocial intervention and behavioral management strategies, including sleep hygiene and avoidance of common triggers such as substance use. Evidence-based psychosocial interventions include group therapy, cognitive-behavioral therapy, and family-focused treatment. IGT is now an evidence-based intervention for maintenance treatment of bipolar disorder and co-occurring SUDs (Weiss et al., 2007, 2009).

SUBSTANCE USE DISORDERS

SUDs (including disorders involving alcohol, drugs, or both) are highly prevalent. In 2009, nearly 22 million Americans age 12 and older (9% of the population) had used an illicit drug during the previous month, and nearly 60 million Americans age 12 and older (about 24% of the population) reported *binge drinking* (defined as drinking five or more drinks on one occasion) during the previous month (Substance Abuse and Mental Health Services Administration, 2010).

As stated earlier, the lifetime prevalence of SUD is approximately six to eight times higher among persons diagnosed with BD compared with the general population (Kessler, Crum, et al., 1997; Regier, Farmer, et al., 1990). This common clinical co-occurrence led to the development of IGT for patients with BD and SUDs. In this section we define SUDs, discuss heterogeneity of the course of SUD, and review current theories about etiology. We also provide a brief review of evidence-based treatments, including group therapies for SUD.

Defining Substance Use Disorder

SUD is defined in DSM-IV-TR (American Psychiatric Association, 2000) by two categories, *substance abuse* and *substance dependence*, distinguished by severity of substance use and extent of loss of self-control over substance use.

Substance abuse involves a problematic pattern of substance use that either results in negative consequences (e.g., family or legal problems) or threatens to do so (e.g., by driving while intoxicated). Substance abuse typically is characterized by some degree of impairment of vocational or academic functioning or difficulties at home. If someone meets criteria for *substance dependence* (described below), then that person cannot also have a diagnosis of substance abuse.

Substance dependence is a syndrome characterized by some or all of the following phenomena:

1. *Loss of control over use* (e.g., a person goes out with the intention of having one or two drinks but has substantially more by the time the drinking episode is over). The lack of control over use may be accompanied by recurrent resolutions to stop or to reduce substance use, sometimes with periods of success followed by recurrences of use.

2. *Increasing preoccupation with substance use.* Increasing preoccupation can be manifest behaviorally in several ways. As drug and alcohol use becomes increasingly important to a person, more time is spent in substance-related behaviors, often to the exclusion of alternative activities. To some extent, the severity of one's substance use can be gauged by the types of activities that are reduced or given up as the result of substance use. For example, milder forms of substance dependence may result in a constriction of non-drug-related recreational activities, whereas increasingly severe substance-related problems may cause people to miss work as a result of their substance use, perhaps lose their jobs, and use drugs or alcohol in situations that are clearly detrimental to their health.

Individuals who meet criteria for substance dependence cannot also meet criteria for substance abuse; the former diagnosis supersedes the latter. Formal diagnostic criteria for substance abuse and substance dependence can be found in the DSM-IV-TR manual (American Psychiatric Association, 2000).

Although these categorical definitions of substance abuse and dependence have clinical utility in assessing the need for specific treatment interventions (e.g., medical detoxification for substance dependence) and/or the urgency of treatment to prevent medical or social risk (usually greater with dependence), the distinction between substance abuse and substance dependence has several limitations when applied practically to individuals or populations of substance users, due to heterogeneity of substance use patterns and risks that may be substance-specific. For example, the injection of opioid drugs or cocaine carries a high risk of accidental overdose and death whether use is infrequent or frequent; likewise, the risk of death is significant for drunk drivers regardless of the pattern and frequency of their alcohol use when not driving.

Individuals with co-occurring psychiatric disorders, including BD, may be at greater risk of harm from any substance use due to both the direct effects of substance use on mental status and the indirect effects of substance use, such as medication nonadherence or drug–medication interactions. In these populations, the distinction between "abuse" and "dependence" may be even less clear, and the distinction may not be meaningful. Since relatively small amounts of substance use may be more harmful in individuals with psychiatric illness than in others (Goldstein, Velyvis, et al., 2006), IGT stresses the desirability of abstinence from substance use, regardless of whether the patient has substance abuse or dependence.

Causes of Substance Use Disorders

The risk for developing an SUD is multifactorial; trends in SUDs differ across substance, gender, and social and regional contexts. Factors that increase SUD risk include family history of SUDs, environmental exposure and access to substances of abuse, early age of first substance use, absence of caregiver monitoring of childhood activities, peer use of substances, lack of knowledge about SUD risks or perceptions of low risk associated with substance use, school dropout and/or conduct problems, lower educational or socioeconomic status, mental illness, stress and negative life events, certain physical illnesses (especially those associated with physical disability, multiple procedures, and chronic pain), cultural acceptance of substance use, ethnicity that predisposes to substance use via heritable and/or cultural factors, antisocial and other deviant attitudes and behaviors, and—for certain substances—gender and/or sexual orientation. It is notable that women are at higher risk compared to men of experiencing SUD-related medical and social consequences early in the course of an SUD, a phenomenon that has been referred to as a *telescoping* course (Hernandez-Avila, Rounsaville, et al., 2004).

SUDs are heritable; genetic risk factors include both nonspecific vulnerability to SUD (i.e., a common risk for developing any SUD) and specific vulnerability to certain substances, such as nicotine or alcohol dependence (Edenberg, Dick, et al., 2004; Kendler, Myers, et al., 2007; Palmer, Young, et al., 2009). Genetic risk factors appear to be influential at all stages of addiction, including initiation of substance use, continuation of substance use, and progression to substance dependence (Li & Burmeister, 2009).

While genetic factors can confer vulnerability, SUDs require initiation of substance use for their expression; even someone at high risk (e.g., with two alcohol-dependent parents) will not develop alcohol dependence without ever drinking. The prevalence of substance use and abuse increases with age during adolescence and peaks in young adulthood. During adolescence, there are minimal gender differences in substance use; however, this changes by young adulthood, such that men are more than twice as likely as women to be diagnosed with an SUD (Palmer, Young, et al., 2009).

Neuronal activity in the brain is altered with all phases of SUD behavioral expression, which can be divided into three aspects of the behavioral cycle of SUD: (1) preoccupation and anticipation of substance use; (2) substance use and intoxication; and (3) withdrawal, which is associated with aversive psychological and physical states that motivate a return to drug-seeking behavior and renewal of the addictive behavioral cycle (Koob & Le Moal, 1997). Changes in brain activity associated with SUDs involve abnormally high activation of brain reward systems leading to pleasant or euphoric subjective states, and abnormal activation of stress response systems leading to unpleasant subjective and physiological states (Koob, 2009). The chronic nature of SUDs may in part be explained by conditioned learning that becomes part of a person's permanent memory. Environmental contexts and internal states (thoughts, feelings, and physical states) that are present during substance use or withdrawal can become learned memories that trigger activation of substance craving and addictive behaviors even during prolonged abstinence from substance use (Feltenstein & See, 2008).

Environmental influences that also affect the likelihood of development of SUDs include availability and cost of the substance, social and legal prohibitions, religious and cultural mores, and familial influences.

The Natural Course of Substance Use Disorders

Recent research evidence supports multiple subtypes of SUDs, with variability in natural course and outcome. Possible manifestations include (1) episodic "binge" use and abuse, (2) a single episode of dependence, (3) multiple intermittent episodes of dependence, and (4) chronic and unremitting dependence. SUDs also show significant variability in age of onset, family history, co-occurring psychopathology, and functional consequences (Hasin, Stinson, et al., 2007; Moss, Chen, et al., 2007). While many individuals meeting criteria for substance abuse and dependence do not seek treatment and recover on their own, those having severe substance dependence typically experience a chronic, relapsing course characterized by compulsive drug seeking and use, and progressive loss of social and behavioral functioning. These individuals ordinarily require treatment interventions to arrest the progression of illness and maintenance treatment to sustain abstinence.

Regardless of whether they are episodic and remitting or chronic and relapsing, SUDs are frequently associated with significant medical consequences. These include infectious diseases such as HIV/AIDS, tuberculosis, hepatitis B and C, cellulitis, pneumonia, and endocarditis (infection of the heart valve); gastrointestinal disease, including pancreatitis; liver disease, including hepatitis, cirrhosis, and liver failure; stroke; high blood pressure; seizures; loss of motor coordination; heart failure; and death by accident/injury or due to organ failure or respiratory depression. Additional medical consequences of SUD-related neuropsychiatric syndromes include depression and suicidality, anxiety, hallucinations, and memory disturbance.

Furthermore, SUDs are associated with a high burden of social, financial, and legal disability. Common examples of SUD-related disability include personal isolation, loss of gainful employment, loss of driver's license, divorce and/or loss of child custody rights, domestic and nondomestic violence, criminal activity to sustain substance use, incarceration, and homelessness.

For both males and females of all ages, and virtually all substances of abuse, SUDs increase the risk of death by accident, injury, suicide, and violence; hence, the detection of risky behavior involving substance use and the prevention and treatment of SUDs is a public health and social priority.

Treatment

There are three primary goals of SUD treatment: (1) an explicit goal to reduce or abstain from substance use; (2) reduction in the frequency and severity of substance use episodes; and (3) improvement in psychological, social, and adaptive functioning (Kleber, Weiss, et al., 2007). SUD treatment is delivered in a variety of settings: inpatient care, residential programs, partial hospital or day treatment programs, intensive outpatient and routine outpatient clinics, integration with psychiatric care or routine primary health care, specialized substance abuse treatment clinics, sober houses, halfway houses, therapeutic communities, peer-support settings (e.g., Alcoholics Anonymous [AA], Narcotics Anonymous [NA], or Self-Management and Recovery Training [SMART] Recovery meetings), community and faith-based settings, employee assistance programs (EAPs), college- and school-based programs, homeless outreach programs, and prison and drug court systems.

SUD treatment recommendations are prioritized by consideration of an individual's medical safety and social functioning; to be successful, the actual interventions are typically negotiated with the individual and implemented according to the individual's stated preferences. Four main principles of SUD treatment are (1) preventing progression of substance use, (2) avoiding imminent and severe medical or social consequences related to the SUD, (3) promoting abstinence, and (4) maintaining abstinence or reductions in substance use. These are briefly discussed below.

Preventing Progression of Substance Use to a Substance Use Disorder

Many substance-using individuals receive their first medical education about the risks of substance use from their primary care clinician or pediatrician. Active screening and brief education, advice to stop using substances, and referral to treatment or support groups (e.g., AA) can be very effective in early intervention and prevention efforts, with sustained reductions in substance use and improvements in multiple functional domains observable at 6-month follow-up (Babor, McRee, et al., 2007; Madras, Compton, et al., 2009).

Avoiding Medical and Social Consequences Related to Substance Use Disorder

People frequently enter SUD treatment after experiencing a negative consequence of their substance use. Initial assessment involves screening for (1) the need for medical detoxification from the substances used, (2) the need to treat SUD-related medical illnesses or injuries, (3) the presence of acute SUD-related neuropsychiatric syndromes and/or suicidal ideation requiring acute stabilization for safety, and (4) the necessity of removing the individual from his or her environment to successfully interrupt the SUD cycle or to avoid SUD-related social consequences. An individual is then directed to an appropriate level of care and setting to receive acute treatment services, followed by arrangement for longer-term continuing care designed to help him or her avoid future dangers of continued substance use.

Promoting Abstinence

For at-risk individuals, those with risky patterns of substance use, and those with SUDs, the safest medical goal is to promote abstinence from all substance use. Multiple interventions are used to support this goal, including early education and public awareness campaigns, motivational interviewing to build an individual's commitment to abstinence, assertive community outreach and reinforcement of abstinence behaviors, and social facilitation through family education and peer-support groups (e.g., AA, NA, or SMART Recovery). In addition, several medications are approved by the Food and Drug Administration to help patients stop substance use, including disulfiram, naltrexone, and acamprosate for alcohol dependence; methadone, buprenorphine, and naltrexone for opioid dependence; and nicotine replacement therapies, bupropion, and varenicline for nicotine dependence. These medications can be used effectively in conjunction with medications for BD in patients with these two disorders.

Maintaining Gains in Reduction of Substance Use

Patients with SUDs, especially severe substance dependence, often require maintenance treatment to prevent relapse to substance use, similar to the way patients with other chronic diseases (e.g., diabetes and hypertension) require maintenance treatment for sustained good health. Maintenance treatments for SUD may include (1) professional treatments in the form of individual or group therapy, family or couple therapy, and medication management; (2) peer-support and self-help groups such as AA and NA, SMART Recovery, and faith-based recovery groups; and (3) structured residential programs that support a recovery environment.

Group Therapy for Substance Use Disorders

Group therapy is the most commonly provided professional SUD therapy intervention. Therapeutic components of group treatments for SUD include the provision of a structured approach, including skills building to maintain abstinence; social facilitation through mechanisms of accountability to group peers and leaders, peer support, and sometimes confrontation of denial and minimization or other relapse behaviors; role modeling of successful abstinence; active and collaborative problem solving among group members; and sustained support and empathy among group members. Group therapy should provide members with an environment that is both safe and confidential; for some individuals with SUDs, this may be a respite from home or other social environments fraught with chaos or conflict.

Although multiple different types of SUD group therapies exist (educational, skills-based, 12-step facilitation, interpersonal, psychodynamic, and check-in groups), most studies have not found differences in efficacy between groups based on specific theoretical models (Weiss, Jaffee, et al., 2004). As described elsewhere in this book, however, a series of studies has demonstrated the efficacy of IGT for patients with co-occurring BD and SUDs. These studies have shown that IGT produces better outcomes with this population than standard group drug counseling.

INTEGRATED TREATMENTS AND INTEGRATED GROUP THERAPY

As stated earlier, many clinicians and researchers have long advocated an integrated approach to the treatment of patients with SUDs and coexisting psychiatric illness. However, there is no single agreed-upon method to accomplish this goal; no "gold standard" characterizes what an ideal form of integrated treatment should be. Rather, integrated models have been developed for patients with schizophrenia, personality disorders, posttraumatic stress disorder, and depression, among others (Kranzler & Tinsley, 2004). These models have provided integrated treatment in a variety of ways. Strategies include alternating between sessions focusing on psychiatric issues and on substance use issues, providing intensive case management, and stressing the importance of medication adherence. IGT integrates the treatment of SUDs and BD in specific ways that we described below.

The Single-Disorder Paradigm

Rather than telling patients that they have two distinct disorders, each of which needs its own treatment, IGT encourages patients to think of themselves as having, in essence, a single disorder called "bipolar substance abuse." The treatment for this disorder involves abstaining from drugs and alcohol; taking medication as prescribed; and engaging in a variety of other "recovery behaviors," such as getting a good night's sleep, recognizing and avoiding situations that present high risk of relapse to either substance use or mood problems, and attending SUD and BD self-help groups. While some recovery behaviors and their underlying thought patterns are specific to one disorder or the other (e.g., learning alcohol and drug refusal; taking mood-stabilizing medication as prescribed), many behaviors (e.g., getting a good night's sleep) facilitate recovery from both disorders. A concrete example of the way the "single-disorder" paradigm is implemented occurs in the "check-in" at the beginning of each group session (described more fully in Chapter 4). Each patient is asked, "Did you use any drugs or alcohol this week? How was your overall mood? Did you take your medication as prescribed?" The check-in thus illustrates the equal weight that each disorder receives, and the manner in which the single-disorder paradigm integrates the treatment of the two disorders.

A Focus on Commonalities in the Two Disorders during the Recovery and Relapse Process

A major theme of IGT is that there are many similarities in the process of recovery from and relapse to BD and SUDs. Thoughts and behaviors are thus labeled in IGT as either "recovery thoughts/behaviors" or "relapse thoughts/behaviors." Commonalities between the two disorders are then discussed. An example of a relapse thought, for instance, is "may as well" thinking ("I may as well stay in bed all day"; "I may as well get drunk"). This is contrasted with the corresponding recovery thought "It matters what I do" ("It matters if I go to an NA meeting"; "It matters if I take my medication"). As described earlier, IGT does not merely focus on recovery or relapse thoughts and behaviors that are specific to BD (e.g., taking medication as prescribed) or SUDs (associating with drug-free friends). Instead, whenever possible, analogous thought and behavior patterns that are relevant to the *other* disorder are raised by the leader, in keeping with the "single-disorder" (bipolar substance abuse) paradigm. For example, the abstinence violation effect ("I've slipped, so I may as well give up and have a full-blown relapse"; see pp. 35–36) is presented as an example of "relapse thinking." An analogous thought process in patients with BD is then discussed ("I'm depressed even though I've taken my medication as prescribed, so I may as well quit taking medication altogether"). The thought pattern behind the abstinence violation effect is thus subsumed under the broader category of "may as well thinking," which is in turn an example of "relapse thinking."

A Focus on the Relationship between the Two Disorders

The third way in which IGT integrates the treatment of the two disorders is by focusing on the relationship between BD and SUDs. Substance use is seen as a risk factor for return to BD and vice versa. Many patients have difficulty accepting the idea that they have two disorders, particularly if they have had more serious consequences from one disorder than from the other. A patient who has been hospitalized many times for BD but has experienced fewer adverse consequences from substance use may find it easier to abstain from cocaine by viewing this as part of the treatment for BD ("Using cocaine is one of the worst things you can do for your bipolar disorder").

How Well Does Integrated Group Therapy Work?

We have now conducted three separate studies of IGT, all of which have demonstrated its effectiveness (Weiss, Griffin, et al., 2000, 2007, 2009). In the first study (Weiss, Griffin, et al., 2000), we compared patients who received IGT to patients who did not receive this new treatment. Like the IGT patients, the latter group received their usual treatment, and both IGT and the non-IGT patients were assessed monthly to examine their substance use, mood, and overall functioning. All patients in this study, and in all subsequent studies we have conducted, had to be taking a mood stabilizer to enter the trial; it is important to note that *IGT is designed to be used in conjunction with medication, not instead of medication.* Moreover, many of the patients in our trials engaged in either individual therapy or case management (Weiss, Kolodziej, et al., 2000). IGT is not designed to replace these, but it can serve as an excellent complement to these clinical services. A total of 45 patients entered this study; most had bipolar I disorder (meaning that they had experienced mania in the past), and most had both drug and alcohol dependence.

Results of this study were highly encouraging for IGT: drug use among the 21 patients receiving IGT decreased from an average of 10 days per month at study entry to an average of less than 1 day per month at the end of treatment. At a follow-up visit held 3 months after treatment was completed, IGT patients continued to use drugs on average for less than 1 day per month. The 24 patients who entered the non-IGT comparison group, in contrast, had much less substantial declines in drug use, from an average of 8 days per month at study entry to 5 days at the end of treatment and 7 days at the 3-months posttreatment follow-up. Alcohol use among IGT patients dropped from 14 days per month on average to 1 day at the end of treatment and 3 days at follow-up. For non-IGT patients, however, alcohol use on average was 7 days per month at study entry, 2 days per month at the end of treatment, and 5 days per month at follow-up. When we examined rates of total abstinence in the two groups, we found that 67% of IGT patients maintained abstinence for 3 or more consecutive months, three times the rate of non-IGT patients (22%). Interestingly, mood improvement was less substantial for IGT; although there was a significantly greater improvement in manic symptoms for the IGT patients, there was no significant difference in improvement in depressive symptoms.

As a result of the encouraging results in this first study, we conducted a randomized controlled trial comparing IGT to Group Drug Counseling (GDC; Weiss, Griffin, et al., 2007). GDC was chosen as a comparison group for IGT because it is designed to approximate the kind of group treatment that would ordinarily be delivered in a community SUD treatment program. GDC is structured similarly to IGT (i.e., with an initial check-in and a session topic); however, GDC focuses primarily on substance use, not on mood. For example, although the "check-in" format is similar in IGT and GDC, the latter differs importantly, in that patients do not report their overall mood for the week, nor whether they took their medications as prescribed; these are important components of the IGT check-in.

This study provided excellent evidence for the efficacy of IGT: IGT patients used drugs or alcohol on approximately half as many days as GDC patients during the trial, although, as in our first study, there were no differences in mood episodes between IGT and GDC patients. Thus, IGT outperformed standard, well-conducted GDC. Still, several obstacles to widespread adoption of IGT in SUD treatment programs remained. First, we realized that the 20-week treatment could be unwieldy for many community programs, because third-party payers, such as managed care companies and state funding agencies, often will not authorize 20 sessions of a treatment. Rather, these payers frequently will authorize 12 sessions of psychotherapy before requiring justification for more visits. To make IGT more accessible to community programs, we thus reduced IGT to 12 sessions. This was not particularly difficult, because our initial version of IGT was in fact 12 sessions; we had initially expanded IGT to 20 sessions in our first study because some of the patients in the 12-session IGT group felt that more treatment would be helpful. But as we describe below, patients did quite well with 12 sessions. Moreover, in a community program that is not part of a research study, patients can stay in the group as long as they find it helpful, and they are not restricted to 12 weeks of treatment.

A second barrier we identified in transferring IGT to community programs was the fact that the group leaders in the first two studies had substantial experience and knowledge about BD and/or CBT. In contrast, many counselors working in community SUD programs have had no formal training in CBT and know little about BD. We therefore modified the IGT manual to include some information about cognitive-behavioral principles and BD. These modifications led to a new question, however: Would 12 sessions of IGT, performed by counselors without training in CBT and without BD experience, still outperform GDC? In our third study we set out to answer that question.

We conducted another study comparing IGT to GDC, using front-line drug counselors without training in CBT or a great deal of knowledge about BD (Weiss, Griffin, et al., 2009). Another modification we made in this study was to conduct IGT as an "open" group, meaning that patients could enter at any time and leave after 12 sessions. The group sessions thus cycled rather than running in a strict sequence in which patients must attend a previous session to acquire the knowledge necessary to attend the current session. We chose an open group format, because this is typically used in clinical settings in which new patients enter a group and others leave on a regular basis. In summary, then, we made three "community-friendly" modifications to IGT, with the idea that if it was successful again, it would be ready for adoption in community programs.

The results of this third study were again very successful for IGT. First, we found that counselors without training in CBT or experience with BD could perform IGT (the version included in this manual) very well. Second, the study showed that IGT patients were nearly three times more likely to abstain from drugs and alcohol completely during all 3 months of treatment (36% vs. 13%) and were more likely to attain at least 1 abstinent month (71% vs. 40%). Moreover, for this study, we developed a measure of what we called a *good clinical outcome*, which we defined as abstinence and no episodes of mania or depression in the last month of treatment. We found that IGT patients were more than twice as likely as GDC patients to be both abstinent and to have no mood episodes in the last month of treatment (45% vs. 20%). These results were highly encouraging. Not only were SUD counselors able to deliver this 12-session version of IGT with favorable outcomes for substance use but improvement was also seen in mood episodes.

Adoption of IGT Elsewhere

With the publication of our results and oral presentation of IGT at a variety of scientific meetings, other programs have begun to adopt IGT for either clinical use or other studies. IGT has been modified for use in a study of patients with both BD and schizophrenia, and has been used clinically in a number of programs in both the United States and Canada. We have spoken with program directors who are using IGT elsewhere, and many of them have made slight changes in IGT to fit their particular circumstances. Some programs have made IGT sessions longer;

indeed, one program runs IGT for 2 hours, with a 15-minute break in the middle. Others have added a parallel program for family members. Some programs have patients read the "central recovery rule" aloud; others have developed "IGT-readiness" groups for patients who are not yet able to achieve maximal benefit from IGT.

We have thus now shown that IGT is an effective treatment for patients with BD and SUD that can be performed successfully by clinicians with different levels of experience and training. IGT can be adapted to meet the needs of specific treatment programs and is enthusiastically accepted by both clinicians and patients. For programs with a sufficient number of patients with these two disorders, IGT can offer an excellent evidence-based treatment approach.

CHAPTER 2

⊙⊙⊙⊙⊙⊙⊙⊙⊙⊙⊙⊙⊙⊙⊙⊙⊙⊙⊙⊙⊙⊙

General Principles of Integrated Group Therapy for Co-Occurring Bipolar Disorder and Substance Abuse

IGT for patients with BD and SUDs is a 12-session group therapy designed for adult men and women with this combination of disorders. This relapse prevention group is designed to attend simultaneously to BD (i.e., through some cognitive-behavioral techniques and a focus on medication adherence) and substance use (focusing on the desirability of abstinence as the safest option for overall functioning and for mood stability). The therapist's main task is to facilitate these two goals by (1) educating patients about the deleterious interactions between the two disorders; (2) tying together themes that are common to the recovery and relapse/recurrence process for both disorders; and (3) emphasizing the "central recovery rule" of IGT, which is described below. Patients are introduced to the concept that their BD and SUDs effectively "blend" into a single disorder (called *bipolar substance abuse* in IGT), for which the optimal treatment includes medication adherence and abstinence from all substances of abuse.

MAJOR GOALS OF THE GROUP

The major goals of IGT are to (1) promote abstinence from drugs of abuse, including alcohol; (2) promote adherence to medications prescribed for BD; (3) teach people to recognize early warning signs of mood difficulties, for the purpose of both sustaining mood stability and SUD relapse prevention; (4) teach social skills that facilitate SUD relapse prevention (e.g., drug refusal skills, avoidance of high-risk situations) as well as mood stability (e.g., prioritizing protective routines such as good sleep hygiene over high-risk social behavior); and (5) improve other aspects of life functioning, including interpersonal relations.

21

As with many of the issues dealt with in this group, it is important to balance different considerations when thinking about these goals. For example, although abstinence is certainly the ultimate substance-related goal of the group, some patients—perhaps a majority of patients—will not be abstinent early in the group. It is important that the therapist be clear about the goal of abstinence, without being critical of patients who do not abstain. Improvements should be noted and new goals collaboratively formulated. For example, an appropriate therapist intervention might be to say, "Mr. X, last week you used drugs on 6 days, and this week you only used on 3 days; maybe next week will be even better," with a facilitated review of the skills the patient used effectively on those sober days.

One of the major foundations of the group is what we call the *central recovery rule*, which is *"No matter what, don't drink, don't use drugs, and take your medication as prescribed—no matter what!"* It is important to remember that, as a whole, this group of patients is discouraged about prospects for recovery. Many have been refractory to treatment, some have given up on themselves, and many have rationalized their continued substance use and erratic medication adherence. Having a strict, simply stated guiding principle instills hope, as long as it is tempered by a clearly empathic, open, positive, and upbeat attitude. The patients may ridicule the central recovery rule as overly simplistic ("Are you telling us to just say no?") and may argue that this rule is too rigid and impossible to follow. However, yielding to that argument may be taking an overly "permissive" stance, and is likely to be interpreted by patients as covertly saying to them, "You're really incapable of recovery, so I won't expect much from you." Our experience with IGT has been that patients may discover previously hidden strengths within themselves, and are pleased when this occurs; this builds self-efficacy for recovery. For example, if a patient says that she has used drugs on 2 days during the week (perhaps with a great deal of shame and discouragement), you can say something like, "What did you do on the 5 other days that you didn't do on those 2 days?" This will remind her that she was successfully abstinent for most of the days, and help her to gain a sense of hope that she might not have been able to attain by merely focusing on what went wrong in the 2 days in which she used drugs. Similarly, when a patient brings up a difficult situation that has recently occurred (e.g., being asked by a friend, "Why aren't you drinking?"), you may ask the group, "I imagine some of you have faced similar situations before; what have you done that has worked?" This reminds people that they have had successes in achieving some recovery in the past. This helps people to recall and call upon their own inner capabilities.

THEORETICAL RATIONALE
FOR THE INTEGRATED GROUP THERAPY APPROACH

Patients who are "dually diagnosed" with psychiatric illness and SUD ordinarily receive treatment according to one of three different models: (1) sequential, (2) parallel, or (3) integrated treatment. *Sequential treatment* consists of treating one disorder first and the other disorder later. In general, a sequential treatment approach initially deals with the most acute disorder; patients may then be referred to another facility or program for the treatment of the other, currently less acute disorder. Sequential treatment is most common in inpatient settings. For example, when treating patients who are acutely manic in a hospital setting, relatively little attention may be paid to their substance use. Conversely, treatment of acute withdrawal on a substance abuse unit may include relatively little focus on psychiatric symptoms.

Parallel treatment, a frequently used model for treating dually diagnosed outpatients, consists of treatment in two different settings, with two different sets of clinicians. For example, a patient may receive treatment for his or her mental illness at a mental health center and go to a substance abuse clinic, perhaps on a different day, for addiction treatment. The advantage of parallel treatment is that the staff members at each clinic are generally knowledgeable about the disorder in which they specialize. They may be less knowledgeable and helpful in dealing with the other disorder, however. Indeed, clinicians in mental health clinics and substance abuse treatment settings often have different philosophies of treatment, which they may clearly convey to patients. Staff members in mental health settings may view substance use as "self-medication" that will improve on its own with treatment of the "underlying" psychiatric disorder. Staff members in substance abuse programs may, conversely, view psychiatric symptoms as consequences of substance use, and may label attempts to obtain medical treatment of these symptoms as "drug-seeking behavior." When a patient in parallel treatment talks about his or her "other" disorder, a common response is for the clinician to recommend that the patient talk about that disorder in the other treatment setting. Thus, a drug counselor may respond to complaints of depressive symptoms by attributing them to "part of the disease of addiction," or may say to the patient, "You need to talk about that with your psychiatrist." Thus, the patient is often left with the task of trying to integrate the treatment of the two disorders, which is made particularly difficult by the often contradictory feedback the patient may receive from the two sets of clinicians.

IGT is an example of *integrated treatment*, which has been recommended by a number of clinicians and researchers for the past decade as being superior to sequential or parallel treatment for dually diagnosed patients. The advantage of integrated treatment is that it is delivered by a single individual or group of clinicians who are "fluent in two languages": the languages of addiction and of mental health. Thus, integrated treatment stresses the importance of dealing with both problems simultaneously, and looks for common themes in the illness development and in the course of recovery from both disorders.

COGNITIVE-BEHAVIORAL THERAPY PRINCIPLES UNDERLYING INTEGRATED GROUP THERAPY

IGT uses many principles of CBT but is not *exclusively* a cognitive-behavioral group therapy; it also uses psychoeducational approaches and recommends use of self-help (often called mutual help) groups, many of which are based on a 12-step model. It is useful for IGT group leaders to be familiar with the key principles underlying CBT, however, because many IGT interventions are based on these core concepts.

What Is Cognitive-Behavioral Therapy?

CBT is a widely used evidence-based psychotherapy that focuses on changing maladaptive thoughts and behaviors (Bieling et al., 2006; Hawton et al., 1989). The goal of the therapy is to identify negatively distorted thoughts and beliefs, and to then restructure these thoughts and beliefs to be more realistic and positive. This is achieved through a collaborative effort between the patient and the therapist to examine healthy norms of thoughts, behaviors, and emotional responses, and to set active goals to achieve a desired outcome. Individuals participating in CBT practice what they learn in sessions and use between-session homework practice assignments, until they have mastered more effective patterns of self-awareness, self-care, and other healthy behaviors.

The main theory underlying the mechanism of action of CBT is that a person's thoughts lead to both behavioral and emotional responses. Behavior, in turn, influences a person's thoughts and feelings. CBT takes an active problem-solving approach: by shifting thoughts and beliefs toward a hopeful and positive assessment of one's capacity to set and achieve goals, the behavioral and emotional responses to working through an identified problem will be more adaptive and have a greater likelihood of success. CBT stresses that, in many instances, a person's perception of a situation has a greater role in determining his or her responses than the actual situation. Thus, CBT emphasizes personal choice and one's capacity to select among competing possibilities for understanding and perceiving one's circumstances, as well as the importance of making positive behavioral choices as a means of improving one's quality of life.

Goals of Cognitive-Behavioral Therapy

CBT sessions are designed to teach a set of problem-solving and self-management skills that can be mastered and then independently applied by the patient following completion of therapy. CBT assists individuals with

- Identifying problems and defining personal goals.
- Developing problem-solving skills.
- Effectively applying problem-solving skills through real-life practice.
- Refining problem-solving strategies to be optimally effective.
- Maintaining skills over time.

Assessment in Cognitive-Behavioral Therapy

The initial assessment identifies maladaptive thought patterns and behaviors, and attempts to elucidate their developmental history. The following factors are influential in the establishment of maladaptive patterns:

- *Situation*—certain locations, environments, or surroundings can trigger a problem.
- *Behavior*—behaviors may serve as triggers for negative emotional responses or be associated with other negative behaviors. For example, methamphetamine use may trigger a mood episode; drinking alcohol may lead to cocaine use.
- *Cognition*—thoughts can lead a person to feel or act in a certain way. For example, the thought "I can't do it" may lead to feelings of powerlessness and behavioral paralysis.
- *Affect*—certain mood states can be conducive to creating or exacerbating problems; for instance, feeling irritable or depressed can negatively affect interpersonal relationships.

- *Interpersonal*—perceptions and interpretations of others' behaviors influence one's thoughts, feelings, and behavior.
- *Physiological*—one's bodily functions influence mood states and behaviors. For example, fatigue may negatively distort one's thoughts and feelings, and lead to ineffective behaviors.

Cognitive-Behavioral Therapy Content within Integrated Group Therapy Sessions

Each IGT session has an agenda with a learning objective and homework assignment for skill practice between sessions. Sessions begin with a review of the learning objectives from the prior session and homework review, then proceed to the next subject topic, with its associated skill practice homework for practice-based learning and mastery. IGT uses CBT-based strategies to emphasize the importance of questioning thought patterns associated with substance use, depression, and medication nonadherence and testing alternative, recovery-oriented thought patterns and behaviors. Examples of CBT techniques used in IGT sessions are listed below.

Symptom Monitoring in Integrated Group Therapy

In Session 1 ("It's Two against One, but You Can Win!"), patients are taught a system of "checking in" weekly on core symptoms of BD and SUD (see Handout 1.2, "Monitoring Your Symptoms: How to Check In on Your Recovery"). Patients use five questions to guide their self-awareness of core symptoms and behaviors in the domains of substance use, mood, medication adherence, risky situations and coping behaviors, and adherence to completing weekly skill practice assignments. Symptom monitoring is expanded in Session 6 ("Reading Your Signals: Recognizing Early Warning Signs of Trouble") to encourage daily symptom monitoring of mood instability and increased desire to use substances.

Core Beliefs in Integrated Group Therapy

Core beliefs refer to personal assumptions and ways of viewing the world that influence people's experience of themselves and others. IGT examines core beliefs of hopelessness and helplessness that commonly dominate an individual's perception in depression and addiction; these beliefs frequently lead to worsened depression and substance use (e.g., Session 3, "Dealing with Depression without Abusing Substances" and Session 10, "Recovery versus Relapse Thinking: It Matters What You Do"). Strategies to change these self-defeating core beliefs include teaching cognitive and interpersonal skills, as well as behavioral activation. IGT also introduces group members to two novel core beliefs that are intended to support health and recovery (see Handout 1.1, "Bipolar Substance Abuse and the Central Recovery Rule"). The first core belief emphasizes that BD and SUDs are highly interactive illnesses; to achieve recovery, therefore, it is helpful to view both illnesses as a single, treatable illness called *bipolar substance abuse*. The second core belief introduced is that successful treatment for bipolar substance abuse requires that an individual always take medications as prescribed and always avoid all use of alcohol and drugs, no matter what situation he or she faces. This core belief, called the *central recovery rule*

("No matter what, don't drink, don't use drugs, and take your medication as prescribed—no matter what!") is placed prominently on the bulletin board every week, and is emphasized in each group session.

Connecting Thoughts to Situations, Mood, and Behavior

The therapist teaches the patient to examine the connection between his or her thoughts and emotional responses in different situations, and to observe how these precede behaviors. Patients are taught to identify maladaptive thoughts that lead to negative feelings, and to practice restructuring these thoughts to more realistic or positive thoughts that lead to more adaptive and/or positive feelings, and ultimately to healthier behaviors. Session 2 ("Identifying and Fighting Triggers") introduces the concept that negative thoughts can produce negative feelings that lead to substance use or relapse. Session 3 ("Dealing with Depression without Abusing Substances") devotes an entire group session to helping patients learn to identify depressive thoughts and to understand how these often lead to relapse thoughts and addictive behaviors. This session teaches patients that (1) negative, pessimistic thinking is a core symptom of depression; (2) it is possible to fight against depressive thinking by replacing depressive thoughts with self-care/recovery thoughts; and (3) cultivating self-care/recovery thinking leads to recovery behaviors instead of relapse behaviors, which help to reduce the burden of depression and the risk of substance use.

Thought Distortions and the Use of Evidence Gathering

IGT recognizes that patients with co-occurring BD and SUDs are challenged by the ways in which their illnesses distort their thinking and perception, especially in social situations. Consequences of poor judgment include substance use and deterioration of important relationships. IGT teaches patients to rely on outside sources of information from people they trust (e.g., family, friends, and members of their treatment team) to "check" that their thinking is healthy. For instance, Session 4 ("Dealing with Family Members and Friends") teaches patients to work at understanding both sides of a relationship and to be open to others' concerns about their behaviors. Similarly, Session 6 ("Reading Your Signals: Recognizing Early Warning Signs of Trouble") encourages patients to pay attention when others voice concern about something they are saying or doing; they are taught to use this information to monitor their recovery instead of dismissing others' observations as unimportant. Seeking feedback from others to address distorted thinking about substance use is discussed in detail in Session 5 ("Denial, Ambivalence, and Acceptance").

Skills Training and Behavioral Problem Solving

Skills training and problem-solving emphasized in CBT are consistent components of IGT. Patients are expected to progress from defining problems to figuring out potential solutions for these problems, and to test these potential solutions in group sessions and through working on the skill practice assignments between sessions. Patients are encouraged to choose the problem-solving strategies that work best for them as individuals, then maintain and implement these skills and problem-solving strategies in the future. All IGT sessions introduce new coping skills and incorporate a skill practice homework assignment to assist the patient's recovery. Sessions with high emphasis on skills training include Session 2 ("Identifying and Fighting Triggers"), Session 3 ("Dealing with Depression without Abusing Substances"), Session 7 ("Refusing Alcohol and Drugs: Thinking It Through and Knowing What to Say"), Session 8 ("Using Self-Help Groups"), Session 9 ("Taking Medication"), Session 10 ("Recovery versus Relapse Thinking: It Matters What You Do"), Session 11 ("Taking Care of Yourself"), and Session 12 ("Taking the Group with You").

Cognitive-Behavioral Therapy in Group Settings Facilitates Peer-to-Peer Learning

CBT can be utilized in an individual setting or in a group; IGT uses the group setting to take advantage of the benefits of sharing experiences among group members. A group can provide an optimistic setting for recovery, since it would be unusual for all group members to be struggling at the same time: the positive example of one member's success or progress can inspire other members who may be having more difficulty meeting their personal goals. Sharing a common problem (e.g., having co-occurring BD and SUD) in a group setting reduces members' feelings of isolation and shame. Participants can also learn from each other and elicit support from other group members. For example, one patient said at a check-in, "I stopped my medication this week. Can people in the group convince me to start taking it again?" In this instance, group members used their own experiences (disastrous consequences from having stopped medication in the past) and IGT concepts such as the "central recovery rule" to persuade him to restart his medication. The homework review can also foster this group process as members give corrective feedback or positive reinforcement to each other. Important therapeutic aspects of IGT groups include the following:

- *Instillation of hope*—the achievements of one group member can inspire others. IGT's emphasis on the possibility for change gives individuals hope that they can work on their problems, alone and together.
- *Universality*—learning that others are suffering from the same or similar problems results in members' feeling less isolated. Hearing how others have managed similar problems is a helpful learning experience for group members.
- *Imparting information*—receiving advice from others in the group, as well as the therapist, gives individuals new information about managing their problems and achieving their desired goals.
- *Altruism*—individuals feel good about giving advice and helping others. Group members in IGT help each other to learn new ways to practice the skills taught in each session.
- *Imitative behavior*—individuals can learn from the behavior of other members. An IGT patient who sees how implementing a new skill has helped another group member may be more motivated to try implementing this skill as well.
- *Group cohesion*—acceptance, support, and trust among group members foster rehabilitative learning. The more cohesive the group is, the more individuals are likely to feel secure in learning from each other.

CHARACTERISTICS OF THERAPISTS

Ideally, a therapist for this group should have completed a certified training program for the treatment of both SUDs and psychiatric illness, and should also have at least 1 year of supervision by a senior clinician, working with patients with co-occurring SUDs and psychiatric disorders. The therapist should also have been supervised in conducting group therapy and should be familiar with relapse prevention concepts, as well as self-help groups available in the local community. The therapist's work should be characterized by warmth, openness, and friendliness, without violating boundaries. The therapist should not be judgmental, harshly confrontational, or condescending toward patients.

We have thus far conducted three successful studies of IGT, using different types of therapists. In the first two studies, we selected therapists who had experience treating both psychiatrically ill patients and those with SUDs. Therapists in these two studies were also familiar with concepts of CBT. After we found in our first study that IGT was enthusiastically embraced by patients and could be delivered successfully by therapists, our second study demonstrated that IGT led to better substance use outcomes than did standard GDC (a manualized, evidence-based treatment focusing primarily on substance use issues and designed to resemble a high-quality version of group treatment as it would ordinarily be delivered in a community substance abuse treatment program). We realized, however, that many substance abuse treatment programs do not have clinicians with mental health treatment experience or proficiency in CBT. We therefore conducted a study to see whether substance abuse counselors without cognitive-behavioral training or substantial mental health experience could conduct IGT successfully. The answer was "yes": we found that experienced substance abuse counselors who were skillful in leading groups, and who met the personal characteristics described earlier, could be trained to conduct IGT successfully.

We have not yet examined whether therapists who are familiar with the treatment of BD but have little experience with SUD treatment could also conduct IGT successfully; this is an open question. The available evidence, however, suggests that expertise in the treatment of substance abuse, skill and supervised experience leading substance abuse and/or dual-diagnosis groups, and an empathic, warm professional attitude are ingredients for success in conducting IGT.

CHARACTERISTICS OF PATIENTS: THE ROLE OF HETEROGENEITY

It is important to realize that a group of patients with BD and co-occurring SUD is heterogeneous in a number of ways depending on (1) the severity and duration of their BD; (2) the severity and duration of their SUD; (3) the level of premorbid functioning and the level of interference with that functioning as the result of the co-occurring disorders; (4) the potential for rapid change in clinical condition that can occur in individual patients from one group session to the next; and (5) the level of acknowledgment of illness and motivation for treatment of one or both disorders. For example, a patient with BD who has experienced stable mood for several weeks may become hypomanic for 2 weeks, then be severely depressed for several weeks. These changes in mood state from week to week can significantly alter the patient's capacity to judge the need for treatment or to apply IGT skills. Moreover, patients may continue to abuse substances, or may build up periods of abstinence. As a therapist, you must therefore be able to adjust the content and level of the group, depending on the clinical condition of the group members. It is important that you do not present the group with content that is too complex for some patients or too simple for better functioning patients. Rather, it is useful to maintain a balance that keeps all patients engaged. Remember that even though some patients may have extremely high levels of premorbid and interepisode functioning, it is critical that they grasp the relatively simple guiding principles (e.g., the central recovery rule) of the group. For patients who object to the simplicity of some of the concepts, it is generally a mistake to make things more intellectualized and complex. Rather, you can say to such patients, "Most of the really important concepts of this group are in fact really simple. For example, nothing could be simpler than the central recovery rule. Usually, when you try to make these ideas more complicated, you're trying to talk yourself into something that you shouldn't, and you're only going to get yourself into trouble."

Although IGT has been designed primarily to treat individuals with an SUD and BD, it has also been adapted in some treatment centers to include individuals with psychotic disorders, including schizophrenia and schizoaffective disorder. This adaptation appears to have been quite successful; patients with these disorders have accepted IGT enthusiastically, and therapists have found that the core principles of IGT are generalizable to psychotic disorders as well. IGT can be used equally well for patients with bipolar I disorder and bipolar II disorder, although the vast majority of people treated with IGT have had bipolar I disorder. Similarly, drug-dependent patients and those with alcohol dependence who have never used drugs can be treated together successfully in an IGT group.

ARE THERE PEOPLE FOR WHOM INTEGRATED GROUP THERAPY IS NOT APPROPRIATE?

IGT was designed to treat people who have a diagnosis of BD and an SUD. As described earlier, other groups of dually diagnosed patients have also been successfully treated with IGT. However, some people are not well-suited for IGT. First, patients who are acutely manic or hypomanic to the degree that they cannot participate meaningfully in a group session without interrupting should not be in IGT. Such individuals are unlikely to benefit from the group because of their difficulty focusing, and they will detract from the experience of other group members. This is a temporary exclusion criterion, however; when someone who is hypomanic or manic attains mood stability, that person may be perfectly appropriate for IGT.

A second exclusion criterion has to do with level of acceptance of one's illnesses. IGT is not particularly helpful for people who absolutely believe that they do not have BD or do not have a substance abuse problem; such individuals are described in the "stages of change" model as being in the "precontemplation" stage, sometimes referred to as *denial*. Anyone in the "contemplation" (*ambivalence*) stage or beyond would be appropriate, however. As long as there is some semblance of belief that the person *may* have these disorders, IGT can be useful.

One of the most difficult clinical situations to deal with is the lack of motivation. Although patients entering IGT must have some desire for this treatment, motivation for treatment of one or more disorders may wax and wane. For example, a patient who is highly motivated to abstain from drug and alcohol use after a crisis may rethink that position after the crisis has subsided. Similarly, a patient whose motivation for treatment of BD is very strong during a period of increased symptoms (e.g., severe depression or an acute manic episode) may change his or her mind when better stabilized. The cognitive-behavioral focus of IGT includes paying a great deal of attention to motivation and to ambivalence. Moreover, the focus on simple rules, such as the central recovery rule, which are repeated frequently, helps to address these concerns consistently throughout the treatment. In addition, patients are reminded at every group session to continue to discuss issues that come up in group with their therapists, doctors, and other recovery supports (e.g., sponsor, self-help peers, friends, or family members) between group sessions.

DISCHARGING SOMEONE PREMATURELY FROM INTEGRATED GROUP THERAPY

Unfortunately, some people who enter IGT need to be discharged prematurely from the group because of their negative influence on other group members. The primary reason for discharging a patient from IGT is that he or she has interfered with other patients' treatment; this may include threatening behavior toward the group leader or another group member, drug dealing within the group, stalking, or any other type of behavior that makes other group members feel unsafe or otherwise interferes with their recovery. In our experience conducting IGT, such events have been extraordinarily rare. Nonetheless, it is important that the group leader protect the therapeutic atmosphere of the group, even it means discharging one of the members prematurely.

DEALING WITH SLIPS AND RELAPSES

Dealing with slips and relapses within IGT should be done in a manner that promotes learning both for the patient who has slipped/relapsed and, equally important, other patients. As described earlier, the therapist should help the patient to understand the behaviors and thoughts that led to the relapse, and distinguish these from behaviors and thoughts the patient had during periods of recovery, even during that week. Asking other patients to try to link the thoughts and behaviors to the subsequent substance use is also very helpful, as long as the therapist is careful to modulate patient feedback so that it fosters neither denial ("It seems as if you couldn't help yourself from drinking") nor guilt and shame ("You really blew it this time"). An example of a statement that avoids these two positions would be, "If you could do that over again, what might you have done differently?"

Recurrences of mood symptoms may be handled similarly, with a focus on whether these episodes are influenced by either medication nonadherence or substance use—both choices within the patient's power to control. An attempt should be made to understand precipitating thoughts or behaviors when they are clear (e.g., feeling that one no longer needs medication, skipping treatment). Sometimes, however, no such clear precipitant exists, and a patient may experience an episode of symptom recurrence (e.g., depression) despite maintaining abstinence from drugs and alcohol, and despite following through completely on his or her mental health treatment. These recurrences are generally the most difficult events for everyone in the group to deal with, since they are required to come to terms with the sometimes vicious nature of BD. Under these circumstances, helping patients to differentiate between those issues they can and cannot control is the task of the therapist, as well as reminding patients of supports available to them through contact with their therapists or case managers, doctors, family, and other recovery supports.

DEALING WITH EMERGENCIES

Occasionally, patients arrive at a group session in a genuine crisis: acutely suicidal, manic, or intoxicated. These patients should be seen individually after the session to assess for crisis stabilization (e.g., hospitalization or 24-hour respite observation).

If some issues warranting serious concern arise during or after the check-in, it is preferable to deal with these as early as possible during the group session, without completely disrupting the session. For example, if a patient expresses suicidal ideation, you should say something like "There is obviously a great deal going on with you right now and you seem very upset. The group setting may not be the best place to talk about all of these issues at this point, but I would like to talk with you about these issues afterward." It is best not to say this during the check-in, since the person's condition may become clearer to you during the remainder of the group. If you are going to see the person individually after the group session has ended, then it is important to let the group members know that you are going to deal with this issue in more depth afterward. This will increase their feelings of safety and their level of confidence in the group and in you. Moreover, they will be able to refocus their energies on the topic at hand, without feeling that this group member will receive insufficient attention.

A patient who enters a group session manic, severely paranoid, or intoxicated can be highly disruptive; having such a person in the group may make meaningful treatment for the other patients impossible. A procedure for handling such emergencies should be in place when beginning IGT. If there are co-leaders for the group, then one leader can step outside the group room and meet with the patient who is experiencing a crisis. Afterward, the group leaders can meet with the patient together to determine the best clinical course of action, including consulting with the patient's psychiatrist. If a patient is hypomanic and thereby prone to speaking too much or out of turn, he or she may be manageable within the group with clear limit setting (e.g., "I think you're a little bit manic right now and I'm going to ask you to hold yourself back from talking, since it's hard for you to focus. Then we can talk individually afterward"). If this type of intervention is successful, it is preferable to isolating the patient from the rest of the group. On the other hand, if you are worried that the patient is irritable and potentially explosive, it is best to have one of the leaders sit with the patient outside the group room. You can say something like "Mr. Jones was clearly having a tough time, and he is seeing Dr. Smith now." Allow patients to talk about their feelings about seeing this patient out of control, and if possible, bring this situation up in the context of the session topic for the day.

CONDUCTING INTEGRATED GROUP THERAPY AS AN "OPEN" OR "ROLLING" GROUP

IGT is designed to be conducted as an "open" group (sometimes called a "rolling" or "rolling admissions" group). This means that new patients can join the group in any given week rather than having all patients begin and end the group cycle at the same time. Because of this, each of the 12 group sessions is presented as a discrete entity, not contingent upon a patient's having attended a previous session. Therefore, if you refer to a concept that was discussed previously, you should be sure to review that concept, so that people who were not present (or who were present but don't recall the concept) understand what you are discussing.

Because each group session is designed to be conducted independently, the order of group sessions is not fixed; rather, it can vary. While the sessions in this manual are numbered from 1 to 12, group leaders should feel free to change the order of the sessions as they feel appropriate to the current condition of the group members. For example, if several people in the group are not taking their medication as prescribed, the group leader might decide to hold the "Taking Medication" session, even if it is not scheduled to be discussed that particular week. Similarly, if a number of patients in the group are experiencing difficulties with family members, then it might be appropriate to conduct the "Dealing with Family Members and Friends" session.

We have run IGT successfully as a "closed" group as well, in which everyone began and ended the group together. Closed groups are logistically difficult to manage, however (see Appendix C: "Frequently Asked Questions about Integrated Group Therapy"), and we therefore recommend running IGT as an open group.

DURATION OF INTEGRATED GROUP THERAPY

This manual comprises 12 different group sessions, each of which is designed to stand on its own. In the research studies we have conducted, patients have received a specific number of group sessions, either 12 or 20, depending on the study, so that we could evaluate the effectiveness of the treatment and compare it to standard group drug counseling in which patients receive the same number of sessions. In clinical practice, using the open group model just described, we recommend that patients' length of treatment with IGT be based on their individual clinical situations rather than attending for a specific number of sessions. Thus, some patients may find that 12 group sessions is the right number for them, but others may find that repeating group topics is helpful. It is often true, for example, that people learn a concept better when they hear it more than once, and it has been our experience when running clinical (i.e., nonresearch) IGT groups that some people find the repetition of these concepts very useful. Since many patients attending IGT are depressed and do not function cognitively at their peak level, they may not be fully engaged in the early sessions, and may therefore benefit from attending more than 12 sessions. If, on the other hand, a patient finds that extra sessions are unnecessary and not valuable, then there is no need to have that person go through the cycle of group sessions more than once.

SESSION LENGTH

In our studies of IGT, group sessions have lasted for 1 hour. We have held hour-long sessions because, in our experience, the attention span of many patients in IGT is relatively short. However, as with many of the other guidelines for IGT, people in other treatment centers have adapted IGT to their own specific patient population. We know of IGT group leaders in some settings that have run 90-minute group sessions successfully, because their patients were able to tolerate that length. Another program we know of has expanded the IGT session length to 2 hours; they spend an hour focusing on the check-in and the skill practice from the previous week, followed by a 15-minute break. The group then spends another hour discussing the current session topic, the session handout, and the upcoming week's skill practice. Thus, IGT is flexible enough to be adapted to the particular setting in which it is taking place.

INTEGRATED GROUP THERAPY VERSUS OTHER APPROACHES

Although IGT is unique in its focus on patients with BD and substance abuse, some elements of the IGT group structure (e.g., the check-in, the use of session handouts) have been used in treatments for other dually diagnosed populations, such as "Seeking Safety," a group therapy for patients with posttraumatic stress disorder and substance abuse (Najavits, 2002). Moreover, some of the topics, such as "Identifying and Fighting Triggers," are standard fare in addiction treatment manuals. What makes IGT unique is not only the particular patient population it treats (those with BD and SUDs) but also the specific method of integrating the treatment of the two disorders: the idea of a single disorder (bipolar substance abuse), the focus on the parallels in the processes of recovery and relapse in the two disorders, and an emphasis on the specific interaction between the disorders.

IGT is based largely on a cognitive-behavioral model. Thus, a great deal of attention is paid to the behaviors and thought processes that promote recovery as opposed to relapse in either substance abuse or mood disorder. For example, the *central recovery rule* ("No matter what, don't drink, don't use drugs, and take your medication as prescribed, *no matter what!*") is described as a recovery-based thought, in contrast to a variety of thought patterns that might lead to substance use or recurrence of mood symptoms (e.g., "It doesn't matter what I do, my life is going nowhere anyway; I'm a more interesting person when I'm using drugs; now that I'm sober, I don't need to take medication").

In addition to focusing on thought patterns, classical (Pavlovian) conditioning is seen in IGT as a major factor in triggering relapse. Thus, there is a good deal of emphasis on identifying and dealing with *triggers* (internal and external cues associated with using substances) in the group. IGT focuses on a combination of (1) identifying recovery versus relapse thought and behavior patterns; (2) learning skills that help to foster recovery (e.g., alcohol and drug refusal); (3) discussing ambivalence about the treatment process itself; and (4) identifying both practical problems (e.g., how to remember to take medication, how to deal with specific side effects, what to say when someone asks you if you want a drink) and emotional difficulties (e.g., depression, feeling rejected by family members or friends).

Although a great deal of attention is paid to level of motivation for treatment (which tends to wax and wane in this patient population), IGT is far more prescriptive than motivational enhancement therapy. For example, the therapist in IGT is clear about the goal of abstinence from substances of abuse and the importance of proper treatment for one's BD. IGT is also not a psychodynamically oriented group. Rather, the group is present- and future-oriented, and does not focus on the role of early relationships in patients' current lives. However, previous episodes of relapse and recovery may be examined in some detail, to the extent that they are instructive in helping people to enter into and sustain a current period of recovery.

IGT is also not primarily a 12-step-based group, although patients are strongly encouraged to attend self-help groups in addition to the therapy group. Indeed, one of the topics in the group sequence is a discussion of self-help groups for people with substance use disorders (e.g., AA, NA, SMART Recovery), mood disorders (e.g., Depression and Bipolar Support Alliance), and for those with co-occurring substance use and psychiatric disorders (e.g., Dual Recovery Anonymous, Double Trouble).

In discussing the treatment of BD in IGT, taking medications as prescribed is viewed as absolutely crucial. Indeed, patients should not enter the group unless they have a prescribing clinician whom they give the IGT therapist written permission to contact. Medication adherence is part of the weekly check-in and is a core concept of the "central recovery rule." IGT also emphasizes the idea that treatment of BD can be further enhanced by (1) coming to a greater level of understanding and acceptance of one's illnesses, (2) understanding triggers for mood symptoms or maladaptive behaviors, (3) understanding recovery versus relapse thought and behavior patterns for bipolar disorder and of course, (4) maintaining abstinence from substances of abuse.

PROSCRIBED THERAPIST BEHAVIORS IN INTEGRATED GROUP THERAPY

As stated earlier, although IGT supports patients' attendance at 12-step and/or non-12-step self-help groups, IGT is *not* a 12-step group. Moreover, IGT is not a psychodynamically oriented group therapy with primarily an interpersonal focus. Therefore, the therapist should *not* do the following:

1. Ask patients when introducing themselves to say, "My name is _____ and I am an alcoholic and an addict."
2. Ask patients to recite the Serenity Prayer in the group.
3. Review specific steps from a 12-step meeting (e.g., "Are you working on your third step?").
4. Focus on interpersonal or transference issues (feelings toward the therapist) within the group, and ways in which these feelings relate to family-of-origin issues (e.g., "You're acting toward me in the same way that you used to act toward your mother").
5. Discuss the relation between childhood issues and current problems.

THE ROLE OF GROUP PROCESS

Although IGT is not a process-oriented group, the relationships among group members and between group members and the therapist certainly affect the character of the group. For example, patients have commented that the "check-in" at the beginning of each IGT group helps them to resist using substances of abuse between group sessions, because they want to report having been abstinent; they don't want to let other group members down. Patients also frequently report that they find the support of other people who have been in similar situations before to be quite beneficial. Group process can, on the other hand, sometimes interfere with the progress of the group. For example, if one or more members are having a particularly difficult time, then this may be discouraging to other group members. In such instances, the therapist must comment on the process to move the group along in a positive direction. However, this is primarily a cognitive-behaviorally based group, and interpersonal relationships should only be a focus if they are interfering with the primary task of the group.

INTEGRATING THE TWO DISORDERS: PUTTING THEORY INTO PRACTICE IN INTEGRATED GROUP THERAPY

How does one integrate the treatment of BD and SUD within the framework of this group? IGT uses three major approaches in integrating the treatment of the two disorders. *First, IGT emphasizes that although patients have two (or more) separate disorders (BD and SUD), these disorders are highly interactive and as such require patients to think carefully about staying sober and following their BD treatment plan faithfully, especially with respect to taking their medications every day.* Patients are taught to think of themselves as ultimately having a single disorder, *bipolar substance abuse,* which is the blending of their BD and SUD, since in effect the problems are so interdependent that they require one primary intervention: medication adherence and abstinence. A variety of other recovery behaviors that are discussed in IGT sessions include skills relevant for the "single disorder" (i.e., getting a good night's sleep; paying attention to one's mood, thoughts, and drug urges; learning to avoid high-risk situations that pose a danger to mood, substance use, or both), and working to improve important relationships with family members and friends. It is thus important to conceptualize that some behaviors and thought patterns promote *recovery* from substance abuse and BD, and others promote *relapse* to substance abuse and *recurrence* of mood episodes. Failure to adhere to one's medication regimen may initially lead to recurrence of mood symptoms, which will place the patient at high risk to use alcohol and drugs. Thus, in IGT, there is no discussion of a "primary" or "secondary" disorder; both disorders are seen as "blending" into a single disorder requiring comprehensive care with pharmacotherapy, abstinence, and psychosocial supports. Treatment for BD is seen as helpful in reducing one's substance use, and vice versa.

A second major approach used in this group is the consistent drawing of parallels between the two disorders. This occurs in several ways. First, the group topics have generally been chosen because they are relevant to both disorders. For example, denial is a common problem in both disorders; Session 5, "Denial, Ambivalence, and Acceptance" is designed to achieve a balanced approach for both disorders. Similarly, sleep difficulties are common among patients with BD and those with SUDs. Therefore, discussing ways to improve one's sleep can help in the treatment of both disorders. Of course, some sessions appear to focus primarily on one disorder (e.g., refusing alcohol or drugs, taking medication). However, even these groups emphasize that these interventions are necessary for the "blended" single disorder of "bipolar substance abuse." Whenever possible, the group therapist actively links the disorders by demonstrating parallels between them, similarities in thought and behavior patterns, and commonalities in treatment principles and the recovery process.

An example of this process occurs in the discussion of the *abstinence violation effect.* This phenomenon, which has been well-described in relation to substance abuse, occurs when someone who has been abstinent for a period of time initially returns to substance use (i.e., violates abstinence). Many such individuals become terribly discouraged and feel like giving up; they may say to themselves, "I've had one drink, so I may as well drink the whole bottle." In IGT, we point out an analogous phenomenon that can occur in patients with BD. For example, some patients who have a recurrence of mood symptoms despite taking their medication as prescribed become extremely discouraged and stop their medication, saying to themselves, "What difference does it make if I take my medication or not?" Whenever possible, the IGT therapist demonstrates the parallels between the sorts of thoughts and behaviors that are necessary for recovery from BD and from SUDs. For example, when a group member talks about experiencing a particular problem (e.g., rejection by a family member) as a result of substance use, it can be helpful for the group leader to say, "Has anyone else had that happen as a result of their bipolar disorder?" This type of question continues to help people understand the link between the two disorders.

Finally, IGT stresses the interaction between the two disorders. IGT emphasizes the impact that one disorder may have on the other. For example, depressive thinking may exacerbate the desire to drink ("My life is hopeless anyway. What difference does it make if I drink?"). Substance use may in turn precipitate a recurrence of mania or depression. Medication nonadherence may cause recurrence of mood symptoms, which may place a person at higher risk for substance use, initiating a vicious downward spiral that frequently results in severe negative consequences, personal losses, and perhaps hospitalization. For some patients whose bipolar disorder may be more severe than their substance use problem (or vice versa), their greatest motivation to abstain from substances of abuse may be the adverse effect of substance abuse on their mood. Thus, a patient whose use of cocaine has not led to serious legal, medical, financial, or family consequences may be persuaded to abstain from this drug because of the fear that cocaine will have a destabilizing effect on BD. Similarly, a patient who is ambivalent about taking a mood stabilizer may be fearful of a manic episode primarily because the poor judgment he or she exhibited during past manic episodes has led to serious relapses to substance use, with resultant personal, medical, or legal consequences.

Therefore, three guiding principles form the core of the "integrated" component of IGT are as follows:

1. BD and SUDs are highly interactive, and in effect "blend" into what can be considered a single disorder.
2. There are parallels between the recovery and relapse/recurrence processes in these two disorders.
3. A clear treatment strategy based on the "central recovery rule" can help improve the outcome of these two disorders (i.e., abstaining from alcohol and drugs, and taking medications as prescribed, no matter what else is occurring in the patient's life).

THE RELATIONSHIP BETWEEN INTEGRATED GROUP THERAPY AND CONCURRENT TREATMENTS

IGT is not a "stand-alone" therapy but is designed to be administered along with other treatment a patient may receive. At a minimum, patients should be receiving medication for their

BD. They may also be receiving pharmacotherapy, when appropriate, for SUDs such as alcohol, opioid, or nicotine dependence. Patients with these co-occurring disorders generally require lifelong pharmacotherapy for their BD, and many need long-term psychosocial supports in addition. Indeed, in the studies we have conducted with IGT, the majority of patients have participated in individual psychotherapy or counseling, in addition to taking medication and attending IGT. In fact, IGT group leaders should actively encourage patients to continue to follow through on the treatments that they are receiving (e.g., meeting regularly with doctors and therapists, attending self-help groups for both the SUD and mood disorders, following through on work tasks, and keeping medical and dental appointments). The therapist should have in advance a signed release of information form to contact the patient's prescribing physician, case manager, therapist, or supporting family member in case of a psychiatric emergency, such as suicidal or homicidal ideation, or an acute worsening of mood symptoms or substance use.

CHAPTER 3

〇〇〇〇〇〇〇〇〇〇〇〇〇〇〇

Therapist Guide for the Integrated Group Therapy Pregroup Interview

It is well known that preparation for group treatment via a pregroup interview can significantly improve the likelihood that a person will attend and be retained in a group. Therefore, the pregroup interview is a critical part of the group process. One of the most important functions of this interview, which typically lasts for approximately 30 minutes, is to get to know the patient as an individual, and to help the patient to feel comfortable with you. Therefore, regardless of the content that is discussed, it is important to establish an open, warm, nonconfrontational, and optimistic tone that will make the patient feel comfortable entering IGT.

Begin by introducing yourself and asking the patient what led him or her to seek out this group. You hope that the patient will talk about problems caused by his or her BD *and* SUD, and specific issues with which the patient would like help. If not, gently ask about other disorders, saying something like "You talked some about your bipolar disorder, but you haven't mentioned anything about drugs or alcohol. Can you talk about what your experience has been with them?" Around this time, ask something like, "What is it that you hope to get from the group?" Assuming that the answer covers something that you believe the group can provide, be upbeat and say, "I think the group can help with that. It's going to take some work on your part and everybody else's, but I think that your goals are perfectly reasonable."

It is important to present a balanced view that you think the group can be helpful, *and* that the group can only work with active effort on the part of the patient and everyone else. Then, review with the patient Handout 1, "Ways to Benefit from This Treatment" (see the end of this chapter). You should ask the patient specifically to identify at least two ways he or she can make the treatment helpful.

You may then ask whether the patient has any special concerns or worries about the group; whether he or she has been in groups before; and whether he or she has particular expectations, hopes, or fears about the group, including topics the patient would like to cover and topics he or she does not want to discuss. You may ask something like

"Is there anything about yourself that you would like me to know that would make it easier for me to help you in the group? For example, some people like to be drawn out if they don't talk much, while some people are worried that they talk too much and appreciate it when someone tries to help them to talk less."

One issue that sometimes arises in IGT is that a patient who is hypomanic (or just overly talkative) may begin to dominate a group. Other group members may become frustrated when such a patient takes over a group; additionally, the patient can become defensive and irritable when cut off by the group leader. The pregroup interview can prepare patients for such an eventuality. It is therefore helpful in the pregroup interview for the therapist to say something like

"One of the things that can happen in this group is that someone may become a little hypomanic and overly talkative. When that happens, if the person happens to be you, I will remind you of this interview. I will say something like 'Remember in our pregroup interview when I said I might cut you off if I found that you were talking too much? Well this is one of those times.'"

By warning patients ahead of time that you may cut them off if they become overly talkative, they are less likely to become irritable and respond defensively when the occasion occurs.

It is important to bring up the issue of dropout very directly. You can say something like this:

"A lot of people with substance abuse problems and bipolar disorder get discouraged if things don't work out well at first. One of the reactions that people may have is to give up and drop out of treatment. If you feel tempted to do this—and you probably will—*don't do it. Thinking* about dropout is perfectly normal, and *talking* about it is a fine idea. But *doing* it is a disaster. This group can't work for you or for anyone else if you don't come; some of the people who have been the most successful are those who have struggled with the idea of dropping out but who haven't done it. This means that even if you are using drugs or alcohol, we want you to come to the group (although we do *not* want you to come to the group intoxicated). The only rule in that regard is that you can't come to the group if you have been using that day. But other than that, if you used the day before or even every day in the past week, I still want you to come. We don't throw people out of the group just because they are using. We want you to learn from your mistakes, and we want you to become abstinent from all substances of abuse."

After this discussion, ask again whether the person has any questions, and answer them. Request that the patient sign releases of information where appropriate, in order for you to be able to maintain contact with members of his or her treatment team (case managers, nurses, and doctors) and, if appropriate, important family members or significant others. Finally, tell the patient that you look forward to seeing him or her at the next group, and say specifically when and where that is. It is important to be upbeat again at this time, as the interview ends.

Ways to Benefit from This Treatment

1. **Come to the group meetings, even when you don't feel like it.** You cannot benefit from this group treatment unless you show up at the sessions. Sometimes, after using drugs or alcohol, or when you feel depressed, bored, or sleepy, you may not want to attend. Come anyway. Also, as part of a group, your absence will definitely affect others (even if you don't think so). You are needed for the group to work for yourself as well as for others.

2. **Participate.** Participation includes listening to others in the group, as well as speaking up, asking questions, and doing the skill practice exercises. By actively participating in the groups, you will get the most out of this treatment.

3. **Be honest.** People with substance abuse problems frequently lie to themselves and to others. Honesty is a key element of recovery. Also, please be honest with the group leader if you have a negative reaction to the group or to a particular session.

4. **Stay focused on your *own* recovery, not others'.** Do not compare yourself to others. You are fighting your own battle; you may be more successful or less successful than someone else in learning something here in the group; you may have more or fewer problems than others in the group. Comparisons at this stage will not help. Just keep trying to do your best.

5. **Be aware that others in the group may be in better or worse condition than you (in either symptoms of bipolar disorder, substance abuse, or both).** The value of a mixed group is that people who are still actively using substances can learn from those who are already abstinent; similarly, people with more severe mood symptoms can learn from those further along in their recovery. If you are further along in either area, it can reinforce your recovery to participate in discussions with people who are at an earlier stage of recovery.

6. **Be aware that the philosophy of this group is to support abstinence from substance use of all types.** To stabilize symptoms of bipolar disorder and help to prevent negative consequences of substance use, it is essential to stop using substances that interfere with stabilization of your mood. Substances of abuse can increase mood symptoms, as well as interfere with the ability of medications to help you with these symptoms. They can also impair your judgment and ability to monitor your mood, and can block your general growth and emotional development. While you may have mixed feelings about giving up substances (a natural reaction at first), it is necessary that you be open to the idea of giving them up.

7. **Complete the skill practice exercises between sessions.** Skill practice exercises are one of the most powerful ways to increase your learning and recovery skills. Not completing skill practice exercises may be a sign of self-neglect (i.e., it can mean that you are not taking care of yourself, not taking the time to do what is necessary to help your recovery).

8. **Recognize the importance of medication in the treatment of bipolar disorder.** For medications to be effective, however, you must be able to take medications as prescribed and to report positive and negative changes to your physician. Central to this process is your ability to monitor your own moods, thoughts, and behaviors; to begin to be able to identify when you might be developing symptoms; and to report this to your therapist or doctor, so that treatment can be adjusted as needed.

9. **Be aware that just as some people have mixed feelings about giving up substances, other people have mixed feelings and/or worries about stabilizing their mood.** Sometimes people worry that stabilizing their mood will decrease their creativity or energy, or replace their good moods with feelings of depression. Moreover, sometimes people find that giving up substances can initially lead to increased depression, especially early in recovery. These symptoms in most cases decrease over time, particularly if you practice the skills learned in the group. Most people who follow the guidelines of this treatment are glad that they did so, because they experience a better quality of life.

I have read the handout, Ways to Benefit from This Treatment. I agree to enter the group and I will try to follow the guidelines discussed in this handout.

From *Integrated Group Therapy for Bipolar Disorder and Substance Abuse* by Roger D. Weiss and Hilary Smith Connery. Copyright 2011 by The Guilford Press. Permission to photocopy this material is granted to purchasers of this book for personal use only (see copyright page for details).

CHAPTER 4

⟨⟨⟨⟨⟨⟨⟨⟨⟨⟨⟨⟩⟩⟩⟩⟩⟩⟩⟩⟩⟩

Conducting an Integrated Group Therapy Session

PREPARING FOR THE GROUP SESSION

Before conducting your first IGT session, we strongly recommend that you read through the entire manual, including all of the sessions, so that you get a sense of the flow of the groups and the nature of the material that will be covered later. By reading through all of the manual material, you gain an understanding of the thinking behind IGT; this will enable you to run much more successful group sessions from the beginning.

Before each session, you should read all of the session material, including the guide for the therapist, the patient session handout, and the skill practice handout. If you have a bulletin board in your group room, we strongly advise you to use it for IGT. Each group session has bulletin board material associated with it, highlighting major themes of that session. In addition, you should always post on the bulletin board the *central recovery rule* ("No matter what, don't drink, don't use drugs, and take your medication as prescribed—no matter what!"). We also suggest that you post the *routes to recovery or relapse* on the bulletin board ("Thoughts → behaviors → relapse or recovery"). Finally, you should post the key elements of the *check-in* on the bulletin board:

1. "Have you used any drugs or alcohol this week? If so, on how many days?"
2. "How was your overall mood during the past week?"
3. "Did you take your medication as prescribed? If not, why not?"
4. "Did you face any high-risk situations or triggers in the past week for either substance use or mood? If yes, how did you deal with them?"

We also suggest that you have a whiteboard and erasable markers in the group room, so that you can write down key points as the group session proceeds. Several of the group sessions involve brainstorming solutions to common problems, and it is important to be able to write these down as they occur.

SESSION STRUCTURE

Each IGT session consists of several core components, each of which should be covered in every group. These core components (with general time guidelines for a 60-minute group; these may be adjusted if resources allow for a 75-minute or a 90-minue group) are as follows:

1. Check-in (and introductions, if appropriate) (15 minutes).
2. Review of last week's group (5 minutes).
3. Review of last week's skill practice (5 minutes).
4. Discussion of the session topic; distribute session handout (30 minutes).
5. Distribute skill practice handout; discussion of skill practice for next week (5 minutes).

Below, we review the purpose of each component and give some guidelines for conducting each portion of the group session.

Check-In (and Introductions, If Appropriate) (15 Minutes)

Key Components of Check-In

Introduce new members, if appropriate, and orient them to the group procedures and central recovery rule ("No matter what, don't drink, don't use drugs, and take your medication as prescribed—*no matter what!*").

Patients then all refer to a "check-in" sequence posted on the bulletin board that prompts them to report on the following questions:

- "Have you used any drugs or alcohol during the past week? If so, on how many days?"
- "How was your overall mood during the past week?"
- "Did you take your medication as prescribed during the past week? If not, why not?"
- "Did you face any high-risk situations or triggers in the past week for either substance use or mood? If yes, how did you deal with them?"

The check-in is a critical part of each group, in which group members report how they are progressing on the major goals of the treatment. Each person's check-in should be generally limited to no more than 2–3 minutes. The check-in establishes the tone for the group. When everyone in the group is doing well, the group is upbeat, optimistic, and generally quite attentive. When many members of the group are doing poorly, as sometimes occurs, pessimism fills the air, and the group members can become discouraged. If only one or two people are doing poorly, other group members are ordinarily quite solicitous and helpful.

It is generally not a good idea to spend too much time exploring in detail how any particular person is doing; however, a *brief* comment after everybody's check-in is helpful, after which you should move on to the next person. *Listen very carefully for check-in reports that can serve as discussion points for the topic of the day, and write these down on the whiteboard as the check-in progresses.* This helps you to organize patient themes for discussion. This can be accomplished as follows:

PATIENT: I had a pretty tough week. I got high 3 days in a row, but I've been able to stay drug-free for the past 4 days. My mood has been pretty lousy and I've been playing around with my medications, taking less lithium than I'm supposed to. I don't really think I did much of any positive coping this week; I know I should have done the skill practice, but I blew it off.

THERAPIST: Well, I'm glad you were able to be drug-free for the last 4 days, but your drug use at the beginning of the week sounds pretty worrisome, and I'm very concerned about your not taking your medication as prescribed. It sounds as though on some days, you were able to achieve some good recovery and do some positive coping, but on other days you weren't. Today we are going to be focusing on denial, ambivalence, and acceptance. Let's have the group help you to think about these things during the topic discussion.

The therapist then may write on the board, perhaps with arrows between indicating interactions: "missed medication → lousy mood → got high earlier in week.

Later in the group, the therapist and group members return to that person's check-in responses and may ask more specifically about how active mood symptoms, missed medications, or environmental triggers might have influenced his or her behavior during the past week; note any connections between these factors and substance use on the board for discussion. In general, it is important to keep in mind the material from the check-in, and bring that into the session topic discussion period rather than focusing on these issues at length during the check-in itself. If some issues warranting serious concern arise in the check-in (suicidal or homicidal ideation, dangerous substance use patterns, psychotic symptoms, etc.), it is preferable to bring up these issues early during the topic discussion, so that the group doesn't feel left in suspense about this person's situation. You may still need to discuss some issues and evaluate them further with the individual after the group has ended. If you decide to take this course of action, you should say so in front of the group (e.g., "I'd like to speak with you for a little bit about some of these issues afterwards"). Don't do this during the check-in, since the person's condition may become clearer to you during the remainder of the group. If you are going to see the person individually, then it is important that the group members know that you are going to deal with these issues in more depth; this increases their feeling of safety and confidence in the group and in you.

After the patients have all checked in, it is a good idea to pull together (using the whiteboard as a visual aid) one or two common themes from the check-in, and to try to relate this to the session topic. For example, if several people have not been adhering to their medication regimens, you might say,

"It sounds as if a number of people are having difficulty taking medication. That issue is at the center of what we are going to be talking about today, since today's group will focus on the process of taking medication. We'll be discussing some of the difficulties you have with taking medications, and how you can cope with those problems."

If people are doing well, it is important to acknowledge that at the end of the check-in. For example, you might say, "It sounds as though people are working very hard, and are taking a lot of the things that they've learned from this group to heart. I think that's great." Increasing the awareness of the group's importance in people's lives can help them to keep the group in mind when trying to decide whether to use substances, take their medication, or enter high-risk situations. For example, people may report that they were abstinent during the week, because they didn't want to "let the group down," or they didn't want to have to report having used substances as part of their check-in. It is therefore important to realize the critical role that the check-in has in a number of patients' efforts to recover.

Review of Last Week's Group (5 Minutes)

After the check-in is over and you have given a brief check-in wrap-up, you should ask people to summarize what they remember from the previous week's group; write the major themes down on the whiteboard. This accomplishes several goals. First, for those who attended the previous week, it establishes a common thread and continuity from one session to the next. Second, people who either missed the previous week's group or had not yet joined the group can learn some of the major principles that were covered the week before. Finally, it can help you as the group leader to see which points from the previous session were important enough for patients to remember a week later. It is helpful to get as many people to participate as possible in this part of the group. As each person brings up a point he or she recalls from the week before, you should write it on the whiteboard. If there are major issues that you think people have forgotten, try to refresh their memories by saying something like "Does anybody remember a discussion we had last week about denial?" If people still don't remember, you should add a couple of points that people do not recall, bearing in mind that this point did not previously make a strong impression on them.

Review of Last Week's Skill Practice (5 Minutes)

Next, you should review the skill practice from last week. You can say, "The skill practice assignment from last week was to write down what you would say if someone close to you offered you drugs or alcohol. How did you find the skill practice? (Wait for some answers.) Who wants to share their answers?" Remind people that the skill practice handouts are an important part of the group; learning and practicing these skills increases their ability to cope. Tell them that this will come in handy when they are challenged with urges to use drugs, not take their medication, or stay in bed all day because of depression. If any patients report during the check-in that they had difficulty understanding or completing the skill practice, address their concerns in the group.

Discussion of the Session Topic; Distribute Session Handout (30 Minutes)

After reviewing last week's session and skill practice, announce the day's topic. Review the main themes of the group session that are listed on the bulletin board (this should take no more than 1 or 2 minutes), then begin the didactic session and discussion. The didactic session and discussion should be combined for most of the rest of the group. When this is finished, distribute and discuss next week's skill practice; this should take about 5 minutes. The didactic material should *generally* follow the patient session handout, but the handout is meant to be a guideline, *not* a specific script. As long as the overall guiding principles of the group are followed and much of the material is covered, it is more important to attend to patients' current issues in relation to the overall topic rather than feeling compelled to cover every detail in the handout.

Since the group will likely be quite heterogeneous in terms of level of education, severity of substance use, and current psychiatric symptoms, it is important to present the material with that in mind. At the beginning of each topic discussion, you can let people know that you realize that you may be discussing material that is familiar to some people but not others. Remember that this is not a class, and that the goal is not to impart as much information as possible. Rather, people should come away with one to three major points from each group they can remember (e.g., "Even if you feel depressed, getting high will make your problems worse" or "Don't depend entirely on your family for your recovery"). Some patients will want you to discuss some topics in great depth (e.g., the neurochemical basis of addiction), while others will find it difficult to follow even the simplest concepts because they are so distracted by their own thoughts. Balancing these extremes can be difficult, and is best accomplished by trying to answer individual questions when it is not too disruptive. Don't forget that simple but critical concepts such as the "central recovery rule" will make the difference between recovery and relapse. Thus, it is important to refer back frequently to major themes such as the similarities between the disorders in recovery and relapse thoughts and behaviors; the central recovery rule; the idea that thoughts lead to behaviors, including relapse or recovery behaviors; the importance of never giving up; the idea of not giving in to relapse thinking; the importance of taking all medications every day as prescribed; the concept that a person can improve his or her recovery by following the treatment plan and working with one's doctor and therapist; and the critical importance of not using alcohol and drugs. Whenever presenting didactic material, try to bring the patients' experiences to the topic, particularly paying attention to what people said during the check-in. Therefore, if the topic relates to the process of taking medication, and a patient has reported during the check-in that she did not take her medication as prescribed during the past week, you can ask her during the didactic session to discuss the thoughts she had about taking medication that led her not to adhere to her regimen that week.

As in the rest of the group, there is a critical balance to be maintained between encouraging people to discuss how difficult it has been for them to recover from their illnesses, while *not* giving them the idea that because recovery is difficult, it can't be accomplished. This balance is difficult to maintain, but it is crucial. It is easy to accept a patient's idea that his life is so terrible that drinking himself into a stupor to escape his misery for an evening isn't a bad option; however, you must be vigilant about empathizing with his pain, while not even *vaguely* agreeing with this way of thinking. Remind people that whatever problems they are experiencing, including depression, will only be made worse by alcohol or drugs. It is important, however, to juxtapose this relatively hard-line behavioral stance with an empathic attitude, recognizing that these patients constantly face an enormously difficult struggle. Indeed, presenting their struggle as a heroic battle against two relentless adversaries (BD and substance abuse) can sometimes invigorate them and make them feel better about themselves.

Whenever possible, it is a good idea to try to get everyone to speak during the didactic/discussion period. One way to do so is to call on someone and say, "You haven't said too much today. Do some of these things we've been talking about relate to you as well?" However, bear in mind that some people in IGT don't speak because they are lost in their own thoughts, and are not really listening. Therefore, don't be surprised if you call on patients and the answers they give are truly off the mark, showing evidence that they have not been attending to the group at all. In this case, try to help the patient save face by briefly discussing that person's concern, then moving back to the topic. By calling on a person, you may be able to reengage him or her with the group, rather than letting the patient drift off for the duration of the session. Furthermore, encourage the peer group to help struggling patients with problem solving. This achieves several goals: (1) It facilitates sharing and discussion within the group, which helps patients to attend to the topic; (2) it promotes self-efficacy by demonstrating that patients are aware of skills to prevent relapse and recurrence of both mood symptoms and substance use; (3) it allows patients to share examples of success they have experienced in controlling their illnesses; and (4) it may facilitate relapse prevention supports between patients outside of group treatment (as patients become more familiar with each other). Write down effective suggestions that patients offer on the whiteboard and review these with the group. Examples of prompting this type of peer facilitation include asking questions, such as "John just said that he keeps drinking because all of his friends drink. Has anyone else in the group ever done this? How can he break this pattern?" Alternatively, you can simply say, "Who can help out John with this problem?"

Session Wrap-Up

With about 8–10 minutes to go in the group, you should distribute and review the session handout as a group and summarize two or three take-home themes that people should try to remember. You might say something like "Okay, we're near the end of today's group. Let's summarize the main points we discussed today that people should keep in mind." Encourage people to state a couple of main points; when this is done, say something like "If you only remember two things from today's group, you should remember the following: that you always need to be on the lookout for denial thinking, and that it's okay to have mixed thoughts about your recovery, but it's not okay to act on them." You should summarize these main thoughts and write them on the whiteboard (in many cases, these will be written on the bulletin board and/or the session handout). Make sure that everybody understands the main points, then move on to the skill practice assignment.

Integrating the Session Handout into the Discussion of the Session Topic

Integrating the session handout into the group can be done in different ways. Some group leaders like to give patients the session handout right after announcing the session topic, while others prefer to give out the session handout only after discussion of the session topic. The advantage of giving out the session handout earlier in the session is that people take in information in different ways; some patients who are able to hear and to read the didactic material simultaneously may retain this information better than they would if they only heard an oral presentation of the material. The risk of giving out the session handout early, however, is that some patients will focus on the written material and not engage adequately in the group. We suggest that you start out by distributing the session handout after announcing the session topic; in general, we have found that this works better. You may want to experiment with giving out the session handout later in the session, to see whether it facilitates a livelier and more engaged group or interferes with the group process.

Discussion of Skill Practice for Next Week

After the group wrap-up, spend 5 minutes distributing and reviewing the skill practice hand-out, making sure that all members understand the content. You might say:

> "Now I'm going to hand out the skill practice for next week. The skill practice for this week is [for example] to write down two ways in which your substance abuse problems and your mood symptoms have negatively affected each other in the past. As we have said before, this group only covers one hour out of 168 hours in the week, so practicing what you learn and talk about here is what's most important. It's very important that you work on the skill practice, then discuss it next week when we meet again. Does anybody have any questions about the skill practice? [Take questions.] Okay. Thank you all very much for coming, and I will see you all next week."

PART II

INTEGRATED GROUP THERAPY SESSIONS

〔⦾⦾⦾⦾⦾⦾⦾⦾⦾⦾⦾⦾⦾⦾〕

It's Two against One, but You Can Win!

SESSION OBJECTIVES

1. Group members will define "bipolar substance abuse" as their diagnosis.

2. Group members will learn a weekly check-in routine that helps them to monitor symptoms of bipolar substance abuse.

3. Group members will be introduced to the *central recovery rule* ("No matter what, don't drink, don't use drugs, and take your medication as prescribed—no matter what!").

MATERIALS REQUIRED

- Bulletin board with the central recovery rule, routes to recovery or relapse, and the Session 1 materials posted.

- Dry erase board and markers.

- Copies of Handout 1.1, "Bipolar Substance Abuse and the Central Recovery Rule."

- Copies of Handout 1.2, "Monitoring Your Symptoms: How to Check In on Your Recovery."

- Copies of Handout 1.3, "Skill Practice Homework Sheet: It's Two against One, but You Can Win!"

51

SUMMARY OF SESSION STEPS AND TIME MANAGEMENT

- **Step 1:** General introductions and group rules (10 minutes).
- **Step 2:** Distribute Handout 1.1. Review the concept of bipolar substance abuse and introduce the central recovery rule (35 minutes).
  - Review symptoms of mania, depression, and substance abuse problems.
  - Teach about ways in which BD and SUDs interact negatively.
  - Introduce the central recovery rule as critical to successful treatment.
- **Step 3:** Distribute Handout 1.2. Review the weekly check-in report and discuss how it relates to the central recovery rule (10 minutes).
- **Step 4:** Distribute Handout 1.3. Review the skill practice for the next group, and congratulate everyone on completing their first IGT session (5 minutes).

BACKGROUND

Co-occurrence of BD and SUDs is common, and is associated with poorer treatment outcomes than having either disorder alone. Many patients will believe that their "real" problem is substance abuse and that the diagnosis of BD is a mistake, or alternatively (and more commonly), that their "real" problem is BD, with their substance use just a form of "self-medication." Patients in this group may even switch between these two ways of viewing their problems, alternately viewing SUD and BD as their "real" or "primary" problem, with the other disorder as either secondary, merely symptomatic of the primary disorder, or nonexistent. Both of these perceptions often interfere with SUD recovery and BD symptom remission. For example, in the first case, patients may readily attend addiction self-help groups such as AA but refuse to take medications necessary to stabilize their mood. These patients will be prone to experiencing depressed, manic, or mixed states, which will increase their risk to relapse to substance use. In the second case, some patients may be willing to take medication prescribed for BD but may continue to use substances because of their impression that their substance use "treats" their mood symptoms more effectively than the prescribed medications. These patients often fail to fully stabilize their moods due to the detrimental effects of SUD on the course of BD. The purpose of this session is to teach patients about the concept of "bipolar substance abuse," which considers the dual diagnosis of BD and SUD as a *single disorder*, with interacting elements of both BD and SUD. Patients are taught that the most effective treatment formula for bipolar substance abuse is (1) abstinence from alcohol and drugs, (2) adherence to medication prescribed for BD, and (3) self-monitoring of symptoms of both disorders.

Step 1: General introductions and group rules (10 minutes).

After the leader(s) introduce themselves, members should say their first names. Leaders then establish the group participation rules. (This is based on Handout 1 in Chapter 3, "Ways to Benefit from This Treatment," which each individual reviewed at the pregroup interview):

"Everyone participating in this group is here because you and/or someone treating you believe that you have both bipolar disorder and substance abuse, and that this combination of problems needs to be dealt with together. You may not see things exactly like your doctor or therapist, but we hope that you will learn effective skills to treat this combined problem that we will call by the name *bipolar substance abuse*. For this group to help you, each of you must pay attention to a few important rules of the group:

1. Come to every group on time, no matter how you are feeling that day. You'll feel better if you do! The one exception to this rule is that we'd prefer that you don't come if you have used drugs or alcohol on the day of the group.
2. Never talk about anything personal that we discuss in this group outside of the group. We must all agree to keep confidentiality—what is said in the group should stay in the group.
3. Keep an open mind and respect each other. Only one person should speak at a time, so that everyone can listen.
4. Be honest. You will not benefit from the group if you are not talking about what is really going on in your mind and your life. We don't judge in this group; we listen and help each other.
5. Please do the skill practice between groups, every week. This will teach you how to apply what you learn in the group. At the beginning of each group, we review the major points of the last group and discuss how you all did with the skill practice. You will learn the most by sharing with each other and practicing on your own."

Step 2: Distribute Handout 1.1. Review the concept of bipolar substance abuse and introduce the central recovery rule (35 minutes).

Review symptoms of mania, depression, and substance abuse problems.

Announce today's topic: "It's Two against One, but You Can Win!" Say that this session focuses on two key concepts that are central to group members. First is the idea that they should think of themselves as having a single disorder called *bipolar substance abuse*. The second point to be emphasized is the *central recovery rule*, which is posted every week on the bulletin board; the central recovery rule serves as a major foundation for the group.

Go to the dry erase board and ask the group members to list symptoms they have experienced during periods of mania. Write down those offered, then compare these to the list in Handout 1.1. Repeat the same exercise for depression and for substance abuse problems, writing the group members' responses on the board. For each category, gather several examples, then compare it to the list in Handout 1.1. Educate and clarify for group members where their personal experiences fit with the handout examples.

Teach about ways in which bipolar disorder and substance use disorders interact negatively.

Next, challenge the group members to think of times when they recall that their mood symptoms led them to drink or use drugs, and list these on the board. Repeat this exercise for times when their substance use was followed by mood symptoms or otherwise interfered with their mental health treatment; list these on the board. As you review these two lists, ask the group whether they think that BD and SUD have any relationship to the other. As they recognize these relationships, introduce them to the concept of *bipolar substance abuse*, a single disorder in which both BD and SUD symptoms interact so closely that it is difficult to know where one begins and the other ends—thus making it easier to view the whole phenomenon as one disorder. Answer any questions that may arise from these discussions, and review the examples that are given in the handout. Ask the group, "Did you know that if you have bipolar disorder, you are more than six times more likely to have a substance abuse problem than someone who doesn't have bipolar disorder?" Educate them on the common co-occurrence of these disorders, and the dangers of not treating both illnesses.

Introduce the central recovery rule as critical to successful treatment.

Finally, introduce the *central recovery rule* by writing this in large letters on the board ("No matter what, don't drink, don't use drugs, and take your medication as prescribed—no matter what!"). Have the group read this rule out loud, and ask for reactions to it. Some members may complain that it is too simplistic or unrealistic. Say to the group, "Even though this rule seems really simple—and it is—it will probably take a while before all of you fully understand how important it is to your recovery. For now, just remember the rule, and we will spend every group session reviewing how to apply this rule every day to help you in your recovery."

Step 3: Distribute Handout 1.2. Review the weekly check-in report and discuss how it relates to the central recovery rule (10 minutes).

Explain to the group members that at the beginning of every group, they will go around the room, allowing each member to "check in" with the group on how he or she is doing with symptoms of BD and with substance use. Tell them that this should only take a few minutes per person and should be kept pretty simple. Review Handout 1.2 to teach them the structure for checking in:

- "Have you used alcohol or drugs since the last group? If so, on how many days?"
- "How was your overall mood since the last group?"
- "Did you take all of your medications as prescribed since the last group? If not, why not?"
- "Did you face any high-risk situations or triggers since the last group? [Briefly explain that these are situations that increase the chances that a person will use, and note that the next group will be focusing on this in more detail.] If yes, how did you deal with them?"

- "Did you complete the skill practice from the last group session? Did you have any trouble understanding it or completing it? Did you go over the skill practice with your doctor, therapist, family, or anyone else?"

Ask one or two members to try checking in with the group for practice, and correct any misunderstandings about the check-in structure and procedure. Encourage the group to think about the check-in questions each day between sessions, since it is very helpful for monitoring progress or problems with bipolar substance abuse. Emphasize *honesty* in checking in. Relate how progress in the check-in report usually corresponds with adherence to the central recovery rule.

With about 8–10 minutes left in the group, you should summarize two or three take-home themes that group members should try to remember. You might say something like, "Okay, we're near the end of today's group. Let's summarize the main points we discussed today that people should keep in mind." Encourage people to state two or three major concepts from today's session; when this is done, you should say something like

"If you only remember two things from today's group, you should remember the following: that bipolar disorder and substance abuse interact with each other, and that it can be helpful for you to think of yourself as having a single disorder called *bipolar substance abuse*. Most importantly, the most effective way to deal with this single disorder is to follow the *central recovery rule*: No matter what, don't drink, don't use drugs, and take your medication as prescribed—no matter what!"

You should summarize these main thoughts and write them on the whiteboard, or point them out on the bulletin board and/or the session topic handout. Make sure that everybody understands these main points, then move on to the skill practice assignment.

Step 4: Distribute Handout 1.3. Review the skill practice for the next group, and congratulate group members on completing their first integrated group therapy session (5 minutes).

Briefly review that the purpose of this session's skill practice homework is to help group members to identify more clearly how bipolar substance abuse affects them individually. Answer any questions the group members have about completing it. Emphasize that the group works best when people complete the skill practice between groups; encourage members to really put effort and thought into it. Let members know that you will discuss the completed skill practice assignments in next week's group. Emphasize that, as a group, they have a lot to learn from hearing each other's experiences and comparing them to their own situation. Tell them that you look forward to seeing them at the next group session.

Bipolar Substance Abuse and the Central Recovery Rule

What are the symptoms of bipolar disorder and substance abuse problems? The major symptoms are listed below. You do not need to have all the listed symptoms to have these disorders, and people may have different combinations of symptoms. What is important is that you learn to recognize the symptoms *you* experience most often. Once you know your patterns, then you can define what "bipolar substance abuse" means to you.

MANIA

Grandiosity (thinking you are very powerful)

Decreased need for sleep

Talking too much or too fast

Racing thoughts (your thoughts are going a mile a minute, faster than you can follow them)

Easily distracted, not able to focus or concentrate

Increased activity level and/or feeling very energetic

Feeling excited or euphoric ("high") about pleasurable activities that will probably lead to painful consequences (e.g., spending sprees, reckless sexual behavior)

Feeling irritable (sometimes people who are manic feel irritable rather than euphoric)

DEPRESSION

Feeling depressed, blue, or down most of the time

Decreased interest in activities, inability to enjoy yourself

Weight loss or gain

Sleep problems (can be trouble falling asleep, waking up in the middle of the night or too early in the morning, or sleeping too much)

Feeling slowed down or easily irritated

Feeling tired or a loss of energy

Feeling worthless or overly guilty

Decreased ability to think, concentrate, or make decisions

Repeated thoughts about death or suicide

(cont.)

From *Integrated Group Therapy for Bipolar Disorder and Substance Abuse* by Roger D. Weiss and Hilary Smith Connery. Copyright 2011 by The Guilford Press. Permission to photocopy this material is granted to purchasers of this book for personal use only (see copyright page for details).

SUBSTANCE ABUSE PROBLEMS

Using drugs or alcohol in larger amounts or for a longer amount of time than you intend (e.g., you intend to have one or two drinks and you end up drinking much more)

A desire or **unsuccessful attempts to cut down**, **control, or stop** your use

Spending a lot of time thinking about drinking or drug use, getting alcohol or drugs, using, recovering from using, or trying not to get caught using

Giving up or reducing family or social activities, job-related activities, or leisure activities because of drinking or drug use

Continued drinking or drug use despite knowing that this causes problems

Tolerance—a need for more of the alcohol or drug to get drunk or high

Withdrawal symptoms when you stop or reduce your substance use

BIPOLAR SUBSTANCE ABUSE

Bipolar substance abuse means that you have symptoms of both bipolar disorder and substance abuse, and *these symptoms interact and make each one even more difficult to control.* Here are just some examples of how bipolar substance abuse is "two against one":

- **Substance use can affect your mood negatively.** For example, heavy drinking can make you depressed; marijuana may make it harder to stabilize your mood; stimulants (like cocaine or amphetamines) can trigger manic episodes; and any substance use can cause problems with sleep, concentration, or thinking.

- **Drinking or using drugs can decrease the effectiveness of your mental health treatment.** These drugs can counteract the effects of your medications and reduce the blood levels of some medications. You are much more likely to miss medications when you are intoxicated. Some people who forget that they have taken their medication may then take too much. Other people who don't take their medication can't remember whether they took it, so they take nothing at all. Often people forget or miss important appointments with their doctor or therapist, just when they need that visit the most.

- **If you don't do everything in your power to treat your mood disorder, severe depression or mania may impair your judgment and may lead you to want to use drugs and alcohol, even if you would not have been thinking that way otherwise.** The hopeless feelings of depression ("It doesn't matter what I do; my life isn't going anywhere anyway") may tempt you to use drugs or alcohol. Even if you understand the negative consequences that substance use brings, these hopeless feelings may convince you that the consequences don't matter.

As you can see by these examples, you are in a battle with two opponents—bipolar disorder and substance abuse—and both are fighting on the same team against you. Your depressive thoughts and your manic symptoms are paving the way for you to return to substance use, and your use of substances worsens your mood disorder. Since the two problems are so closely related to each other, we call the combination of the two disorders bipolar substance abuse. Although you may not have thought of it this way, it is important to realize that if you want to fight either problem, you have to fight them both at the same time. Even if you are much more worried about having another episode of depression than about your substance use, remember that these two forces are fighting together against you. If you return to

(cont.)

57

substance use, you put your mood in danger. Similarly, if you are worried about your substance abuse problem but aren't sure about the need to treat your mood problems seriously, you need to know that getting depressed or manic puts you at great risk for returning to substance use. This is why successful treatment can be boiled down to one formula we call the central recovery rule:

CENTRAL RECOVERY RULE

NO MATTER WHAT,
DON'T DRINK, DON'T USE DRUGS,
AND TAKE YOUR MEDICATION AS PRESCRIBED—
NO MATTER WHAT!

You will learn a lot more about how to live by the central recovery rule in the following group sessions. For now, just focus on remembering the rule. If you learn nothing more from these groups than this rule, you still will have learned the single best tool to stay sober and to maintain good mental health. The rule is so important that you will always see it posted in large letters at every group, and we discuss how to use it at every group session.

Monitoring Your Symptoms:
How to Check In on Your Recovery

You may be wondering, "With so much to keep track of, how can I effectively monitor my progress in recovery from bipolar substance abuse?" This "check-in" procedure is designed to help you do just that. At the beginning of every group, each member takes about 2–3 minutes to give the group a sense of how recovery is going by answering the following **four check-in questions**:

1. Have you used alcohol or drugs since the last group? If so, on how many days?
2. How has your overall mood been since the last group?
3. Did you take all of your medications as prescribed since the last group? If not, why not?
4. Did you face any high-risk situations or triggers since the last group? If yes, how did you deal with them?

As you will see, the check-in helps to keep you on track with how well you are doing with the central recovery rule. It asks you to consider whether you have done well this week with abstaining from alcohol and drugs. If yes, what helped you to accomplish this? If not, what can you learn from it that will help you to do better next week? It also asks whether you have taken your medication every day as prescribed, no matter what else was going on with your mood, thoughts, or daily events. If yes, do you notice feeling better? If you don't feel better, did using drugs or alcohol contribute to this? If you did not take your medications as prescribed, what got in the way? What could you do differently to help you take your medication as prescribed more regularly next week? By checking in on your progress, and on other group members' progress, you will begin to see how the patterns of bipolar substance abuse cause problems for people, and how living by the central recovery rule leads to a better recovery.

From *Integrated Group Therapy for Bipolar Disorder and Substance Abuse* by Roger D. Weiss and Hilary Smith Connery. Copyright 2011 by The Guilford Press. Permission to photocopy this material is granted to purchasers of this book for personal use only (see copyright page for details).

Skill Practice Homework Sheet: It's Two against One, but You Can Win!

Patient Initials: _____

Date: _____

Please write down two ways in which your substance abuse problems and your mood symptoms have negatively affected each other in the past. You might wish to go over these examples with your doctor, your therapist, or someone else important to you.

1. _____
   _____
   _____
   _____
   _____
   _____

2. _____
   _____
   _____
   _____
   _____

Please write down at least one thing you plan to do differently this week that will help to avoid having either of these situations happen again. Ask your doctor, therapist, or someone important to you if they think your idea will work. (You may add more than one idea, if you like.)

_____
_____
_____
_____
_____
_____
_____
_____
_____
_____

From *Integrated Group Therapy for Bipolar Disorder and Substance Abuse* by Roger D. Weiss and Hilary Smith Connery. Copyright 2011 by The Guilford Press. Permission to photocopy this material is granted to purchasers of this book for personal use only (see copyright page for details).

Identifying and Fighting Triggers

SESSION OBJECTIVES

1. Group members will learn to identify "triggers" of substance use (internal or external cues that increase their chances of using substances). Patients will also learn that some triggers (skipping medication doses, staying up all night) can precipitate a mood episode.

2. Group members will be introduced to basic cognitive-behavioral concepts, with emphasis on the possibility of changing relapse thoughts and behaviors to recovery thoughts and behaviors.

3. Group members will review common types of triggers: those that are dangerous for most people (e.g., seeing someone else drinking or using drugs) and those that are specific or personal (e.g., hearing music that the patient used to listen to while taking drugs).

4. Group members will learn that substance use is a trigger for mood destabilization, while bipolar disorder symptoms are triggers for substance use.

5. Group members will learn the *AAA method* for managing triggers: *avoid* triggers when possible, don't face triggers *alone*, and engage in a distracting *activity* or get *away* when triggers are present.

MATERIALS REQUIRED

- Bulletin board with the central recovery rule, routes to recovery or relapse, and the Session 2 materials posted.
- Session 2 bulletin board material.

- Dry erase board and markers.
- Copies of Handout 2.1, "Identifying and Fighting Triggers."
- Copies of Handout 2.2, "Skill Practice Homework Sheet: Identifying and Fighting Triggers."

SUMMARY OF SESSION STEPS AND TIME MANAGEMENT

- **Step 1:** Check-in procedure (15 minutes).
- **Step 2:** Review last week's group topic, "It's Two against One, but You Can Win!" and ask group members to explain the meaning of "bipolar substance abuse" and the "central recovery rule" (5 minutes).
- **Step 3:** Review last week's skill practice questions on Handout 1.3, "Skill Practice Homework Sheet: It's Two against One, but You Can Win!" (5 minutes).
- **Step 4:** Distribute Handout 2.1. Introduce the concept of "triggers" for substance use and mood problems, and introduce the AAA method for managing triggers (30 minutes)
  - Triggers can be people, places, objects, feelings, or thoughts that make a person want to use alcohol or drugs. Triggers also can start a mood episode (missing medications, poor sleep patterns, or unstructured days).
  - Introduce the idea that thoughts lead to feelings and behaviors.
  - Ask the group members to identify things that trigger their desire to use drugs or alcohol, or make them begin to feel depressed or manic.
  - Triggers can be external (people, places, and things) or internal (thoughts and feelings).
  - Instill optimism.
  - Fight triggers using the AAA method.
    - *Avoid* triggers when possible.
    - Don't face triggers *alone*.
    - Distract yourself from triggers by getting *active* or getting *away*.
  - At the end of the session, summarize with a discussion of the major points.
- **Step 5:** Distribute Handout 2.2. Tell group members to practice using the AAA method this week (5 minutes).

BACKGROUND

Many patients attending this group experience their mood episodes or substance use as events that "happen" to them; they often feel that they have no control over these phenomena. This group is designed to teach patients that they are not powerless over their illnesses, and that learning more about actively managing their illnesses will enable them increasingly to feel a sense of control over their illnesses rather than having the illnesses control them. The idea of developing and practicing active skills to maintain good health and sobriety is conveyed to reinforce the central recovery rule, which should be reviewed at every group session.

The group leader will introduce the concept of a *trigger*, which is defined as any external cue (e.g., people, places, things) or internal cue (e.g., thoughts and feelings) that increases the chances that a person will want to use alcohol or drugs. It is also emphasized that some situations can trigger a mood episode. Moreover, using substances is frequently a trigger for depression or mania, while symptoms of depression or mania can serve as triggers of substance use. Although triggers will always be present to some degree, group members can improve their recovery by learning to use the AAA method for dealing with triggers (*avoid* triggers where possible, don't face triggers *alone*, distract yourself from triggers by getting *active* or getting *away* from them).

Step 1: Check-in procedure (15 minutes).

Following the group leader's announcements (e.g., expected member or leader absences, changes to the group meeting schedule or site), all patients should review their weekly progress according to the Handout 1.2, "Monitoring Your Symptoms: How to Check In on Your Recovery (see Session 1). During this time, other group members are discouraged from commenting on the individual's check-in report, since relevant discussions can occur during the review of the skill practice. The group leaders should make brief summary comments that provide recognition and positive reinforcement for any changes in thoughts or behaviors that indicate group members are making efforts to achieve abstinence and mood stability or to apply the central recovery rule. The check-in is also a time for the group leaders to listen carefully for any content that might provide a useful opportunity for the group to discuss this week's group topic; here, leaders note on the board patients' reports of triggers of substance use or mood instability, focusing on how the members did or did not make an effort to manage them.

Step 2: Review last week's group topic, "It's Two against One, but You Can Win!" and ask group members to explain the meaning of "bipolar substance abuse" and the "central recovery rule" (5 minutes).

Try to get as many members of the group to participate in this as possible, checking to ensure that they grasp the core concepts about the interactions of the two disorders. Write the main points of the previous group on the dry erase board. Sometimes, group members may not readily recall the main points of the prior session. In this situation, refresh their memories by asking prompting questions, such as "What effect does using substances have on symptoms of bipolar disorder? Can bipolar disorder symptoms be related to substance use? How?"

Step 3: Review last week's skill practice questions on Handout 1.3, "Skill Practice Homework Sheet: It's Two against One, but You Can Win!" (5 minutes).

Elicit group volunteers to review their responses to last week's skill practice. Positively reinforce their efforts to apply what they learned in the group. If any members did not complete the skill practice, review with them content in their check-in that might pertain to that skill practice. Alternatively, invite them to answer one or more of the skill practice questions in the group, if they are able to do so. Highlight any examples in which members' completion of skill practice questions appears to have helped them to report good progress at their check-in.

Step 4: Distribute Handout 2.1. Introduce the concept of "triggers" for substance use and mood problems, and introduce the AAA method for managing triggers (30 minutes).

Triggers can be people, places, objects, feelings, or thoughts that make a person want to use alcohol or drugs. Triggers also can start a mood episode (missing medications, poor sleep patterns, or unstructured days).

Start out by stating the session topic—"Identifying and Fighting Triggers"—and say why this topic is important, namely, that *triggers consist of people, places, things, feelings, or thoughts that increase the desire to use substances.* Then add, "For people with bipolar disorder, a trigger can also be something that makes it more likely for you to have symptoms of depression or mania, like missing medication or not getting enough sleep." You should say that some people refer to triggers as *high-risk situations,* although the actual term used is not particularly important. Why do triggers exist? Explain that the brain stores memories of people and circumstances associated with using substances, or associated with episodes during which a person feels depressed or manic. Even after you get sober, or get better after a mood episode, those memories are still there, and they can be reactivated—or "triggered"—by new people or events that remind you of past times using substances or feeling depressed or manic. Thus, triggers are cues that make you think about your past experiences of using substances or feeling depressed or manic, and these thoughts can sometimes make you *feel* like you did during a substance abuse or mood episode. If you feel like using, you're at greater risk for using. If you feel depression creeping in, you're at greater risk for experiencing a full-blown depressive episode again.

Introduce the idea that thoughts lead to feelings and behaviors.

This is a good time to *introduce basic cognitive-behavioral concepts* and to write these on the board, stating,

> "In this group we will talk a lot about how thoughts can lead to behaviors, so that changing your thoughts can be a way to avoid or change risky or otherwise unhealthy behaviors. Also, changing your behaviors can have a big impact on your thoughts and feelings. For instance, applying the central recovery rule and choosing to be abstinent and to take your medications will have a positive impact on your mood and feelings, and will lessen depressed thinking. These are ideas that we will be talking about at every session, since these ideas are the building blocks for your recovery skills."

Ask the group members to identify things that trigger their desire to use drugs or alcohol, or make them begin to feel depressed or manic.

Ask questions such as "What are your triggers for substance use?", "What are your triggers for depression?", and "What are your triggers for mania?" Write down their responses on the board in three columns: one each for substance use, depression, and mania. After you have several responses, begin to show how some triggers are common to most people, such as watching someone else get drunk or high, seeing the substance you used to use, or seeing a person you used to drink with. Then point out or ask for other triggers that may be more specific to the individual: a birthday or anniversary, a certain situation, a song on the radio, a specific person or relationship. Tell the group, "Everybody has both common and specific triggers. If you learn to identify what triggers you, you will have the power to avoid or to control these triggers, so that they don't control you."

Triggers can be external (people, places, and things) or internal (thoughts and feelings).

Now, make two columns on the board for listing *internal* and *external* triggers for substance use. Explain that internal triggers are thoughts, feelings, or physical states that trigger urges to use; that external triggers are people, places, things or events outside of us that trigger urges to use. Ask group members to suggest a few examples for each column. The list in their session handout is below:

Internal	External
Sadness, anger, loneliness	Someone hurts your feelings or makes you angry.
Negative thoughts	Someone tells you that using is fun.
Physical discomfort	Someone offers you drugs or alcohol.
Positive thoughts about using	You see something that reminds you of using.

While reviewing examples of substance use triggers, emphasize that *drug and alcohol availability is typically the single factor most likely to increase the desire to use.* Even if you are not thinking about getting high, seeing your drug of choice may suddenly and dramatically cause you to want the drug. The safest path is to avoid being around drugs and alcohol, so that you don't use.

A final point to emphasize is that *substance use can be a trigger for making mood symptoms worse, and mood symptoms can be a trigger for relapse to substance use,* even if the person is not aware of these associations at the time. Some group members may offer personal examples to illustrate this point.

Instill optimism.

Before getting into the details of how to fight triggers, it is important to instill optimism in the group that they can be fought. Many people in the group have been unsuccessful in previous attempts to fight off the desire to use substances, and have been paralyzed by depressive feelings. Therefore, the idea that triggers and high-risk situations can be fought successfully is a new one, and group members are likely to be quite skeptical of the idea. Begin by asking, "Has anyone in the group ever successfully avoided or fought off a trigger?" Find out from them what has worked in the past, and write one or two examples from the group on the board.

Fight triggers using the AAA method.

- AVOID triggers when possible.
- Don't face triggers ALONE.
- Distract yourself from triggers by getting ACTIVE or getting AWAY.

After this, bring up the "AAA method" of fighting triggers. As defined in Handout 2.1, AAA stands for:

- *Avoid* the trigger when possible.
- Don't face triggers *alone*.
- Distract yourself from triggers by getting *active* or getting *away*.

Ask the group, "What are some triggers that you think you *can* avoid, and what are some that you think you *can't* avoid?" Distinguish between situations that are *difficult* to avoid versus those that are *impossible* to avoid. Challenge group members to come up with solutions for avoiding certain situations that may be difficult, but not impossible, to avoid. Next, discuss triggers that cannot be avoided completely, but that one can avoid facing *alone*. Ask people to describe certain situations that fit this category, and refer to the session handout for examples. A useful discussion may involve being invited to parties or weddings in which alcohol will be served, or which may go very late into the night, disrupting safe sleep routines.

Internal triggers may be especially difficult to avoid. For example, people may find that when they are home in the evening, they feel lonely and depressed, and want to escape those feelings; perhaps they are disturbed by racing thoughts and want relief from this. Remind the group that using drugs or alcohol in this situation is virtually certain to make those feelings worse rather than better in the long run. These symptoms are best managed by talking to others for comfort and reporting symptoms to one's doctor or therapist. Remind them that connecting to others helps win the fight against triggers: "Don't forget that family, friends, or an AA or NA sponsor can be very helpful for coping with mood symptoms that make you think about using drugs and alcohol."

At the end of the session, summarize with a discussion of the major points.

- Triggers are relatively common, and everyone has particular personal internal and external triggers.
- If you know your triggers, you can plan a strategy to fight against them.
- Triggers are difficult, but they can be fought.
- The AAA method is a successful method of fighting against triggers.

With about 8–10 minutes left in the group, you should summarize two or three take-home themes that people should try to remember. You might say something like, "Okay, we're near the end of today's group. Let's summarize the main points that we discussed today, which you should keep in mind." Encourage people to state two or three major concepts from today's session; when this is done, you should say something like "If you only remember two things from today's group, you should remember the following: It is important to prepare yourself to deal with both internal and external triggers, and the best way to deal with them is with the AAA method." You should summarize these main thoughts and write them on the whiteboard, or point them out on the bulletin board and/or the session topic handout. Make sure that everybody understands these main points, then move on to the skill practice assignment.

Step 5: Distribute Handout 2.2. Tell group members to practice using the AAA method this week (5 minutes).

Encourage group members to pay attention in the coming week to triggers that threaten either their commitment to sobriety or their mood stability. Tell group members that they will have plenty of opportunity in the upcoming week to be on guard for triggers, and that it will be important for them to identify these, then practice the AAA method of dealing with triggers. Next week, when they review the skill practice, they can provide feedback on each others' efforts and give advice on handling difficult situations; fighting triggers is always easier with help from others. End the session by saying that you look forward to seeing them again next week.

Identifying and Fighting Triggers

WHAT IS A TRIGGER?

- A **trigger** is a person, place, or thing that increases your desire to use drugs or alcohol. There are also triggers that can be a mood or a thought, or a feeling of physical discomfort.
- Some triggers may make you begin to feel depressed or manic.
- A trigger can be **internal** (feelings and thoughts) or **external** (people, places, situations, and things).

EXAMPLES OF TRIGGERS

Internal	External
Sadness, anger, loneliness	Someone hurts your feelings or makes you angry.
Negative thoughts	Someone tells you that using is fun.
Physical discomfort	Someone offers you drugs or alcohol.
Positive thoughts about using	You see something that reminds you of using.

- It is important to remember that it is impossible to *always* avoid triggers. However, you should try to avoid them whenever possible. If you *cannot* avoid a trigger, then the goal is to learn to manage your response to the trigger without using alcohol or drugs.
- Be aware that triggers can set you off very quickly and suddenly, so you must always be prepared to fight them off.
- Symptoms of bipolar disorder are often a trigger of substance use. Making sure that you are following your treatment plan and taking all of your medication every day, as prescribed, will help to reduce your mood symptoms, so you will be less likely to use.

FIGHTING TRIGGERS WITH THE "AAA METHOD"

You **can** learn to manage triggers. Practice the three A's:

- **Avoid** triggers when possible.
- Don't face triggers **alone**.
- Distract yourself from triggers by getting **active** or getting **away**.

1. **Avoid** triggers when possible.

   Sometimes it is very *difficult* to avoid a situation, but it is still *possible*. Examples of avoiding triggers include the following:

- Change your route while going home, to avoid passing your dealer's house.
- Get all of the alcohol out of your house, so that you don't have to face it and be tempted by it.

(cont.)

From *Integrated Group Therapy for Bipolar Disorder and Substance Abuse* by Roger D. Weiss and Hilary Smith Connery. Copyright 2011 by The Guilford Press. Permission to photocopy this material is granted to purchasers of this book for personal use only (see copyright page for details).

- Do not go to a party during early recovery if alcohol is going to be served.
- Stay away from people with whom you used drugs or alcohol.
- Avoid situations that have previously triggered mood symptoms, such as staying up too late or not taking your medication.

2. Don't face triggers **alone**.

Sometimes, there is no way you can avoid facing a particular high-risk situation. When you have identified situations that trigger you, a good rule of thumb is as follows: "If you *can't* avoid a high-risk situation, avoid facing it *alone*." For example, if you are concerned about abusing prescription drugs, don't go to a doctor's office alone. Bring someone with you who will make sure that you don't ask the doctor for pain medication to relieve your headaches. Similarly, if you are in the habit of stopping off at a bar on the way home from work, driving to and from work with someone else may help you get over that hurdle early on. Having someone with you won't make it *impossible* for you to return to substance use, but it will make it a little bit more difficult, which may be all that it takes to get you through a risky time successfully.

Being with other people can also help you to deal with feelings of depression. If you're alone with your depressive thoughts, you are likely to sink deeper. Being with other people can be very therapeutic by getting your focus away from negative thoughts and feelings.

3. Distract yourself from triggers by getting **active** or getting **away**.

Any form of activity that can take your mind off of the trigger usually helps. For example, you can distract yourself with self-nurturing activities such as reading, TV, calming music, exercise, taking a walk, going to a movie, or doing a craft or hobby. Keeping busy by having a structured schedule that focuses your attention away from triggers may also be helpful. Activity can also help fight depression. It provides distraction, a feeling of purpose, and can help you fight the sense of paralysis that depression can cause.

SUMMARY

Be aware that fighting triggers, as with any other behavioral change, may feel awkward and uncomfortable at first. Avoiding or resisting triggers almost always creates anxiety, upset, or anger—and it may be that only later will you feel good about having done so. Keep in mind the difference between short-term feelings when trying a coping technique (which may be difficult) and long-term feelings (which will be positive).

Skill Practice Homework Sheet:
Identifying and Fighting Triggers

Patient Initials: _____

Date: _____

1. List one trigger for your substance use.

   _____

   _____

   How do you plan to deal with this trigger successfully?

   _____

   _____

2. List one trigger for depression.

   _____

   _____

   How do you plan to deal with this trigger successfully?

   _____

   _____

3. List one trigger for mania.

   _____

   _____

   How do you plan to deal with this trigger successfully?

   _____

   _____

From *Integrated Group Therapy for Bipolar Disorder and Substance Abuse* by Roger D. Weiss and Hilary Smith Connery. Copyright 2011 by The Guilford Press. Permission to photocopy this material is granted to purchasers of this book for personal use only (see copyright page for details).

Dealing with Depression without Abusing Substances

SESSION OBJECTIVES

1. Group members will understand the concept of depressive thinking and behavior.

2. Group members will identify and share several examples of depressive thinking and depressive behavior, highlighting problems that are common to the group.

3. Group members will identify their own particular manifestations of depressive thinking and behavior, highlighting problems that pertain to their specific situations.

4. Group members will collectively discuss strategies to fight against their depressive thinking and behaviors.

5. Group members will learn that it is necessary to fight against depressive thinking and behaviors, since these can in turn lead to substance use relapse thinking and behaviors.

MATERIALS REQUIRED

- Bulletin board with the central recovery rule, routes to recovery or relapse, and the Session 3 materials posted.

- Dry erase board and markers.

- Copies of Handout 3.1, "Dealing with Depression without Abusing Substances."

- Copies of Handout 3.2, "Skill Practice Homework Sheet: Dealing with Depression without Abusing Substances."

SUMMARY OF SESSION STEPS AND TIME MANAGEMENT

- **Step 1:** Check-in procedure (15 minutes).
- **Step 2:** Review last week's group topic, "Identifying and Fighting Triggers" (5 minutes).
- **Step 3:** Review last week's skill practice questions on Handout 2.2, "Skill Practice Homework Sheet: Identifying and Fighting Triggers" (5 minutes).
- **Step 4:** Distribute Handout 3.1. Introduce the concept of "depressive thinking" and how to cope with it (30 minutes).
  - Demonstrate how thoughts lead to behaviors that can be destructive (relapse behaviors) or positive (recovery behaviors).
  - Depression affects not only feelings but also thoughts. Discuss common types or patterns of depressed thinking.
  - Like relapse thinking, depressive thinking is diseased thinking and not the truth.
  - Introduce common coping strategies to deal with depressive thinking.
- **Step 5:** Distribute Handout 3.2 and encourage everyone to pay attention in the coming week to depressive thoughts or behaviors that could lead to relapse behavior (5 minutes).

BACKGROUND

Many patients in this group feel helpless and paralyzed at the onset of a depressive episode. Frequently, their despondency over being depressed leads them to believe that nothing can be different or better for them, so it doesn't matter if they revert to using substances. Alternatively, they may believe that substance use can give them a reprieve from feeling depressed. On the contrary, substance use tends to worsen the course of depression.

This group session covers a cognitive-behavioral principle, namely, that thoughts can lead to behaviors. The goal of this session is to help people (1) to identify the thinking and behavior patterns that are characteristic of depression (i.e., irrational pessimism, difficulty with priorities, isolation, and inactivity); (2) to distinguish these thoughts and behaviors from the normal course of events; and (3) to fight actively against these cognitions and behaviors rather than using them as a basis for subsequent behavior. The group leader should emphasize the principle of "recovery" thoughts and behaviors versus "relapse" thoughts and behaviors, and try to teach the group how depression can "trick" a person into forgetting or ignoring the central recovery rule.

Step 1: Check-in procedure (15 minutes).

Following the group leaders' announcements (e.g., expected member or leader absences, changes to the group meeting schedule or site, introductions for new members), all patients should review their weekly progress according to Handout 1.2, "Monitoring Your Symptoms: How to Check In on Your Recovery" (see Session 1). During this time, other group members are discouraged from commenting on the individual's check-in report, since relevant discussions can occur during the review of the skill practice. The group leaders should make brief summary comments that recognize and positively reinforce any thought or behavioral changes that indicate that group members are making efforts to achieve abstinence and mood stability or to directly apply the central recovery rule. Check-in is also a time for the group leaders to listen carefully for any content that might provide a useful opportunity for the group to discuss this week's group theme; here, leaders note on the board patients' reports of depressive thoughts and behaviors that may have interfered with their ability to apply the central recovery rule effectively.

Step 2: Review last week's group topic, "Identifying and Fighting Triggers" (5 minutes).

Ask group members to explain the concept of triggers—both for substance use and for BD symptoms. Elicit several examples of triggers, reviewing the differences between internal triggers (thoughts, feelings, subjective states) and external triggers (people, places, things, and events). Review the "AAA method" for countering triggers (*avoid* triggers; don't face triggers *alone*; when faced with a trigger, either get *away* or distract yourself with *activity*). Try to get as many group members as possible to participate in this by inquiring about whether they used the "AAA method," and whether it was difficult. Most group members will indeed report that avoiding and fighting triggers is not easy. You therefore should note on the board any effort in which a person felt discouraged, to elicit supportive feedback from other group members. Remind members that fighting triggers is always easier to do with help from others, and that members can learn a lot from each other in sharing their experiences and asking for assistance with managing high-risk situations.

Step 3: Review last week's skill practice questions on Handout 2.2, "Skill Practice Homework Sheet: Identifying and Fighting Triggers" (5 minutes).

Elicit group volunteers to review responses positively reinforce their efforts to apply what they learned in the group. If any members did not complete the skill practice, review with them any content in their check-ins that might pertain to skill practice questions. Alternatively, invite them to answer one or more of the skill practice questions in the group, if they are able to do so. Highlight examples in which members' completion of skill practice questions appears to have helped them to report good progress at their check-in. Make a special note of any member who reports depressive symptoms as triggers for substance use, stating, "This is such a common experience that we are devoting today's group discussion to the topic of managing depression without using substances."

Step 4: Distribute Handout 3.1. Introduce the concept of "depressive thinking" and how to cope with it (30 minutes).

Demonstrate how thoughts lead to behaviors that can be destructive (relapse behaviors) or positive (recovery behaviors).

Announce today's topic—"Dealing with Depression without Abusing Substances." Start out by asking, "How hard do you think it is to use the central recovery rule when you are depressed?" This will likely elicit multiple responses you can use to illustrate how depression is often manifested by thoughts and behaviors that interfere with self-care and recovery efforts. After writing down a few examples, use the board to illustrate in a flowchart how thinking affects behavior, and how behavior leads to either relapse or recovery. Make sure that every group member understands this cognitive-behavioral principle before proceeding with the rest of the group discussion. Show two examples of a thought leading to a relapse behavior, as opposed to a thought leading to a recovery behavior (you may be able to use material from members' check-in reports for this). Then show how changing the thought that led to the relapse behavior can result in a recovery behavior instead.

Depression affects not only feelings but also thoughts. Discuss common types or patterns of depressed thinking.

Point out that while people typically see depression as affecting mood, it also changes our thinking. Ask group members whether they have any ideas about some of the thoughts that go through their heads when they feel depressed. Typically, patients will describe thoughts of pessimism, negativity, hopelessness, and worthlessness. Write down some of these thoughts on the board. Then you can ask, "If you are thinking this way, how is that likely to affect your behavior?" Encourage group members to describe some of the behaviors that would follow naturally from negative, pessimistic thinking. In particular, you should encourage people to talk about how this might affect their decision whether to use drugs or alcohol. One common pathway might be as follows: A thought such as "I don't care what happens to me. Nothing good will ever happen to me" can easily lead to the next thought, "I may as well get high just to give me a little bit of relief; staying straight isn't going to help my life anyway." This thought can then lead to relapse behaviors. Try to achieve a balance here between focusing on how depression can lead to substance use and other negative consequences, even during periods of abstinence.

Like relapse thinking, depressive thinking is diseased thinking and not the truth.

After reviewing some of the behaviors that might follow from depressive thinking, it is important to emphasize that although these behaviors *can* follow from depressive thinking, they don't *have to* follow. In particular, they don't have to follow if some of the depressive thoughts are identified as such, rather than being identified as realistic commands that need to be followed. *Identify depressive thinking as* diseased *thinking, much like "relapse thinking" in addiction (e.g., "One line of cocaine can't hurt"); emphasize that this type of thinking needs to fought rather than obeyed.* One of the characteristics of depressive thinking that makes it difficult to fight is its "self-righteous" nature. People who are in the grips of depressive thinking don't just *think* that things will always go badly for them. Rather, they are *sure* that nothing will ever work out for them. Therefore, identifying depressive thinking as a problem rather than the voice of truth is critical. One group session is obviously not enough to review all the ways of fighting depression. However, if patients can understand the concept of depressive thinking and begin to identify depressive thinking as a *problem*, they will have accomplished a good deal.

Introduce common coping strategies to deal with depressive thinking.

The next portion of the group focuses on the ways that people can begin to cope with depressive thinking. Ask the group, "Now that you have identified some typical depressive thoughts, what can you do to help yourself when you notice them?" Some of the ideas about coping with depression are listed in Handout 3.1. These include:

- Understanding depressive symptoms so that you can report them to your doctor or therapist.
- Making sure that you do not make things worse by using drugs or alcohol.
- Injecting some self-doubt into the self-righteous depressive thoughts by understanding that they are not reality-based.
- Beginning to fight against depressive inertia and pessimism by tackling some of the tasks that are typically avoided because of depressive pessimism.

An example of this, listed in Handout 3.1, is returning telephone calls. One way to stimulate discussion of this topic is to say, "Tell me about a recent time when you were depressed, and what some of the early symptoms were." Typically, you will hear a story of someone who stayed in bed, let tasks pile up, and angered friends and family members by not following through on commitments. You can then ask whether other people have had similar experiences, and the answer will likely be affirmative. Then ask how people have dealt with their depression under such circumstances. Typically, the answer will relate to climbing out of their depression one step at a time (e.g., returning one phone call at a time, or talking to one friend at a time, and beginning to follow through again on commitments). Try to elicit at least one positive action that each group member has taken to fight against depression. Write down each action on the whiteboard, and end this segment of the session by reviewing the list and pointing out the variety of methods people have used to fight depression.

With about 8–10 minutes left in the group, you should summarize two or three take-home themes that people should try to remember. You might say something like "Okay, we're near the end of today's group. Let's summarize the main points we discussed today that people should keep in mind." Encourage people to state two or three major concepts from today's session; when this is done, you should say something like "If you only remember a few things from today's group, you should remember the following: that depression affects the way we think; that depressive thinking needs to be fought, not obeyed; and that substance use will make your depression worse, not better." You should summarize these main thoughts and write them on the whiteboard, or point them out on the bulletin board and/or the session topic handout. Make sure that everybody understands these main points, then move on to the skill practice assignment.

Step 5: Distribute Handout 3.2 and encourage everyone to pay attention in the coming week to depressive thoughts or behaviors that could lead to relapse behavior (5 minutes).

When group members notice depressive thoughts and behaviors, they should practice one of the skills outlined in their handout (helping your mood, not hurting your mood, changing your thinking, changing your behavior). Tell them to write down examples that can be discussed at the beginning of next week's group. End the session by saying that you look forward to seeing them again next week.

Dealing with Depression without Abusing Substances

Symptoms of depression can feel like a nightmare, with sadness, a lack of energy, an inability to enjoy life, hopelessness, restlessness, and despair. These symptoms can persist in spite of your attempts to get better, and this can create a sense of hopelessness, a belief that things will never get better. You can have depressive symptoms without knowing that you are sick; it might seem that you are unhappy because you deserve to be unhappy, or because you have created a situation that you cannot escape.

Being depressed tends to change your thoughts negatively. The way that you think and the way you feel are very closely related. Therefore, when you feel depressed, it is important to pay attention to your thoughts. Depressive thinking can fool you into believing that your life is worthless or doomed to failure. Depressive thinking can sometimes even trigger negative hallucinations, such as voices telling you that you are worthless or evil, or hopelessly addicted. These negative thoughts can become the basis of behaviors in your life that may lead you to more trouble. By paying attention to the way that you think, and by questioning some of the negative thoughts that often go along with depression, you may be able to move toward recovery.

CHARACTERISTICS OF DEPRESSIVE THINKING

- Depressive thoughts seem realer than real, but they are not real.
- Depressive thinking makes you feel down on everything and everybody, especially yourself.
- Depressive thinking tends to make you stay away from other people, which makes you feel more lonely, isolated, and depressed.
- Being depressed can make your thoughts confused, so that even simple tasks (grocery shopping, taking a shower) feel overwhelming and seem impossible to carry out.
- Since you avoid doing things when you feel depressed, other people (family, friends, employer) may become angry or critical of you. This can make you even more depressed.
- Depressive thinking can sometimes include hearing voices that criticize you or tell you to do self-destructive things.

COPING WITH DEPRESSION

Coping with depression involves making changes on three different levels: your mood, your thinking, and your behavior. While these all work together, it is important that you start somewhere, since improvement in any one of these will begin to help the others.

1. Helping Your Mood

One of the areas always worth examining is whether there is some medication that may be able to help improve your mood. Very often, people who are depressed do not report depressive symptoms to their doctor or other clinician. They are convinced by their depressive thinking that they deserve to have a miserable life, and that nothing can help them; they don't even recognize this as depression. Therefore, it is important to understand symptoms of depression so that you can report them early on. If you are not sure whether you have symptoms of depression, ask your doctor or your therapist about it.

(cont.)

From *Integrated Group Therapy for Bipolar Disorder and Substance Abuse* by Roger D. Weiss and Hilary Smith Connery. Copyright 2011 by The Guilford Press. Permission to photocopy this material is granted to purchasers of this book for personal use only (see copyright page for details).

2. Not Hurting Your Mood

A common problem that people experience when they feel depressed is the wish to "self-medicate" these symptoms with drugs or alcohol. While people sometimes experience a temporary improvement in mood from using alcohol or drugs, they often use these drugs to escape from feelings altogether. Use of alcohol or drugs among people with bipolar disorder and substance abuse problems is not self-medication: it is really **self-poisoning**. It may feel good temporarily, just as sugar tastes good to people with diabetes. However, both are instances of trading temporary good feelings for long-term pain. If you think of substance use as "self-medication," you are much more likely to continue using. You have to change the image of substance use in your mind to one of poisoning yourself, so that you can talk yourself out of it when you are faced with the urge to use.

3. Changing Your Thinking

Having depressive thinking is a little bit like wearing dark glasses, but without being aware that you have on dark glasses. When you wear dark glasses, everything that you see looks dark. Your past looks dark, your present looks dark, your future looks dark, and your relationships look dark—everything looks dark. Whenever someone else attempts to tell you that things aren't so dark, you react by thinking that person doesn't know what he or she is talking about, because the darkness is perfectly clear to you. Since depressive thinking does not tolerate other points of view, the most important thing you can do to begin dealing with depressive thinking is at least to be aware that you have on the dark glasses. Ask yourself, "Would someone else I know be thinking this if he were in my situation? Would I think like this about someone else in my situation?" By "getting outside of yourself" a little bit, you may be able to see that the way you've been thinking about yourself isn't the only possible point of view. Rather, it is a sign that you are experiencing depressive thinking. Try talking to your family, therapist, or doctor about this.

4. Changing Your Behavior

What do you do when you feel overwhelmed, paralyzed by a lack of energy, and convinced that you have 100 things to do, all at once? The first task is to realize that you need to start somewhere, and that having 99 things to do is better than having 100 things to do. If you do nothing, you will soon have 101 things to do, and you will feel even worse. It matters what you do. Therefore, set a priority to get something positive done.

Here's an example that may sound familiar. A common early symptom of depression is not returning phone calls, so that people often end up with 20 phone calls to return and feel overwhelmed. You want the problem to go away—to have no calls to return, but that is unfortunately not an option. The only two options are to take a small step toward recovery, make *one* call, and have 19 left, or take a step backward, and soon you will have 21 calls to return. Therefore, if you have 20 phone calls to return, pick the one call that you find easiest to make. Once you have done that, you will begin to challenge the idea that you can't do anything. Having 19 calls to return is better than having 20, certainly better than 21, and getting yourself going is the most important step. With each small step that you make, the next step becomes slightly easier. Depression often feeds on itself: the longer you do nothing, the easier it is to continue to do nothing. Fortunately, recovery also feeds on itself. Once you get started doing something—*anything*—it gets easier and easier to continue with your recovery.

Skill Practice Homework Sheet:
Dealing with Depression without Abusing Substances

Patient Initials: _____

Date: _____

1. List one depressive thought that you have had.

_____

_____

_____

2. List a way that you plan to deal with this depressive thought.

_____

_____

_____

3. List one depressive behavior that you have had.

_____

_____

_____

4. List a way that you plan to deal with this depressive behavior.

_____

_____

_____

From *Integrated Group Therapy for Bipolar Disorder and Substance Abuse* by Roger D. Weiss and Hilary Smith Connery. Copyright 2011 by The Guilford Press. Permission to photocopy this material is granted to purchasers of this book for personal use only (see copyright page for details).

SESSION 4

Dealing with Family Members and Friends

SESSION OBJECTIVES

1. Group members will understand that difficulties with family members and friends are common; they are more the rule than the exception.

2. Group members will learn how essential it is to recovery that they not use these difficulties as reasons for substance use, medication nonadherence, or other self-destructive behaviors.

3. Group members will discuss how relationships in early recovery frequently get worse before they get better, because the experience of early recovery by substance abusers is entirely different from the recovery experience of their family members and friends.

4. By trying to understand the experiences of family members and friends, and by realizing how different their experiences are from group members' own, it is possible to become more accepting of these differences and less disappointed in these relationships.

MATERIALS REQUIRED

- Bulletin board with the central recovery rule, routes to recovery or relapse, and Session 4 materials posted.
- Dry erase board and markers.
- Copies of Handout 4.1, "Dealing with Family Members and Friends."
- Copies of Handout 4.2, "Skill Practice Homework Sheet: Dealing with Family Members and Friends."

79

SUMMARY OF SESSION STEPS AND TIME MANAGEMENT

- **Step 1:** Check-in procedure (15 minutes).
- **Step 2:** Review last week's group topic, "Dealing with Depression without Abusing Substances" (5 minutes).
- **Step 3:** Review last week's skill practice questions on Handout 3.2, "Skill Practice Homework Sheet: Dealing with Depression without Abusing Substances" (5 minutes).
- **Step 4:** Distribute Handout 4.1. Discuss how thoughts and behaviors related to bipolar substance use can negatively affect relationships, and how to help repair these relationships (30 minutes).
  - Thoughts and behaviors can lead to interpersonal problems.
  - Both sides of interpersonal problems are understandable.
  - Stick to the central recovery rule "no matter what," including during interpersonal conflict.
  - Five ways to help heal relationships:
    1. Follow through on your treatment.
    2. Share your recovery experiences with family members.
    3. Include others in your treatment—this may be a relief for both you and others close to you.
    4. Understand that relationships in early recovery often get worse before they get better.
       - Only the substance abuser knows for sure whether or not he or she is clean and sober.
       - Only the substance abuser knows for sure whether he or she even has any *intention* of remaining clean and sober.
       - Family members often wait to express their anger until their relative has become sober.
    5. Try to see things from the other person's point of view.
- **Step 5:** Distribute Handout 4.2 and encourage everyone to pay attention in the upcoming week to opportunities to help repair relationships that need improving (5 minutes).

BACKGROUND

This session is often one of the most difficult and affectively charged sessions for the group member, since important relationships frequently are strained when a person is actively depressed, manic, or abusing substances. When a person is acutely ill, his or her thinking and judgment may be profoundly impaired, leading to behaviors that are destructive to relationships (overspending, not meeting responsibilities, verbal or behavioral transgressions, sexual indiscretions, illegal behavior, etc.). During early recovery, group members are commonly faced with heavy burdens of negative consequences, shame, and broken relationships—all of which need active efforts to repair. Unfortunately for the individual in early recovery, not everyone is patient and understanding about the wreckage; in fact, most individuals in early recovery have at least one important person who has been hurt badly, and who makes sure to remind them just how much damage they have done. Thus, the purpose of this session is to help group members do the following:

1. Understand better the common difficulties that people with BD and SUDs frequently experience in their relationships with family members and friends.
2. Put their own experiences in perspective, by hearing about other group members' relationship difficulties.
3. Identify ways they can improve these relationships—or, if this is not possible, to cope better with their disappointments regarding relationship difficulties.

Early in this session, it may be helpful to ask a group member to recite the central recovery rule. You then comment,

"The central recovery rule includes a phrase that is so important it is repeated; that phrase is "No matter what!" This means that, no matter how badly you feel during early recovery, no matter who may be giving you grief for poor choices or behaviors while you were sick or using, no matter how embarrassed you may be or how guilty you feel for having hurt someone close to you, no matter *what* anyone says to you, you still need to abstain from using drugs and alcohol, and you need to take your bipolar disorder medications every day as prescribed. If you don't, relationships will go from bad to worse, and you will feel even worse about yourself. But if you stick to the central recovery rule, people will see that you are making a genuine effort to get well and to be responsible, and your relationships with them can improve over time."

Tell group members that this session is meant to help them learn how to manage difficult relationships in a way that will support their own recovery and begin the important process of making amends to others they have hurt because of their bipolar substance abuse.

Step 1: Check-in procedure (15 minutes).

Following the group leaders' announcements (e.g., expected member or leader absences, changes to the group meeting schedule or site, introductions for new members), all patients should review their weekly progress according to Handout 1.2, "Monitoring Your Symptoms: How to Check In on Your Recovery" (see Session 1). During this time, other group members are discouraged from commenting on the individual's check-in report, since relevant discussions can occur during the review of the skill practice. The group leaders should make brief summary comments that recognize and positively reinforce any thought or behavioral changes that indicate that the group members are making efforts to achieve abstinence and mood stability or to directly apply the central recovery rule. Check-in is also a time for the group leaders to listen carefully for any content that might provide a useful opportunity for the group to discuss this week's group theme; here, leaders will make note on the board of members who report problems in relationships that may be affecting their mood negatively or interfering with their ability to apply the central recovery rule effectively.

Step 2: Review last week's group topic, "Dealing with Depression without Abusing Substances" (5 minutes).

Ask group members to give some examples of depressed thinking, depressed behavior, relapse thinking, and relapse behavior. Ask someone to describe how feelings, thoughts, and behaviors are related. Ask members if they believe that a person can change his or her feelings, thoughts, or behaviors to support recovery rather than relapse; write examples of this on the board.

Step 3: Review last week's skill practice questions on Handout 3.2, "Skill Practice Homework Sheet: Dealing with Depression without Abusing Substances" (5 minutes).

Elicit group volunteers to review responses and positively reinforce their efforts to apply what they learned in the group. If any members did not complete the skill practice, review with them any content in their check-in that might pertain to that skill practice's questions. Alternatively, invite them to answer one or more of the skill practice questions in the group, if they are able to do this. Highlight any examples in which members' completion of skill practice questions appears to have helped them to report good progress at their check-in. Make a special note of any situations in which members report conflicts with family and friends that led to depressive thoughts or behaviors, or substance use thoughts or behaviors; ask the group if anyone else has experienced this after an argument with or criticism by a friend or family member. Tell them, "Getting back on track with people that you care for is an important part of recovery, so today we are going to discuss how to begin to do that."

Allow about 5 minutes for this opening discussion to help group members begin to share personal events that are difficult to talk about because they usually involve feelings of guilt, shame, or blame and resentment. Be careful to avoid allowing members to indulge in sharing long tales of interpersonal events; you might interject with "It's pretty clear that everybody has had their fair share of relationship problems that make it tough to stay on track with recovery. So today we are going to talk about how to think about troubled relationships in a way that helps your recovery."

Step 4: Distribute Handout 4.1. Discuss how thoughts and behaviors related to bipolar substance use can negatively affect relationships, and how to help repair these relationships (30 minutes).

Thoughts and behaviors can lead to interpersonal problems.

Announce today's topic: "Dealing with Family Members and Friends." Say that relationship problems are nearly universal in people with BD and substance abuse, and they can be very painful. Say that this session will focus on how to approach troubled relationships in a way that can be helpful to recovery.

Start out by saying, "In the last group, we talked a lot about thoughts and behaviors. In this group, we will continue to do this, because there can be two sources of problems in relationships: problems caused by certain behaviors that are upsetting to another person, and problems caused by certain negative thoughts related to another person." Draw two columns on the board labeled "behaviors" and "thoughts," and ask group members to think of examples of relationship problems they experienced when they were having BD symptoms or actively using substances. If members hesitate, you may be able to use some of the check-in content as beginning examples, or refer to the examples outlined in Handout 4.1.

Both sides of interpersonal problems are understandable.

As you are writing examples on the board, ask members to determine whether they saw the problem as originating with them (in which case the negative consequences likely include feelings of guilt or shame) or with the other person (in which case the negative consequences likely include angry feelings and resentment). Then ask whether anyone can imagine how the other person might have contributed as well. The purpose of this exercise is to *help group members to generate a more balanced view of relationship conflicts—seeing ways in which both sides may be understandable* and both sets of behaviors may create tensions and problems.

Stick to the central recovery rule "no matter what!," including during interpersonal conflict.

No matter how other people treat them, no matter what circumstances they encounter, group members are responsible for their own recovery. This philosophy again harkens back to the "central recovery rule" that no matter what, they must not use alcohol, not use drugs, and take their medication as prescribed—no matter what. In this case, the "no matter what" refers to "no matter how you are treated by people close to you." Say something like

> "Having your spouse leave you is not a reason to use drugs. Being rejected by your family is not a reason to stop your medication. The fact that your mother worries about the people you spend time with or asks you what you plan to do with your money may make you angry, but this does *not* mean that she is driving you to drink or do anything else self-destructive."

These are painful, sometimes devastating events, but giving up on the central recovery rule will only lead them to worse problems.

Five ways to help heal relationships.

The next part of the session focuses on ways that people can help to heal these relationships. The five major categories of activities that can help to heal relationships, which are discussed in Handout 4.1, are listed below. These all involve patients' separating their own recovery from the responses other people have toward them, while allowing family members to participate in their treatment where appropriate (e.g., family members are frequently essential in helping patients to obtain and take prescribed medication properly).

   1. *Follow through on your treatment.* It is important to keep in mind that following through with treatment by no means guarantees that one's relationships will improve signifi-

cantly. However, *not* following through on treatment substantially increases the likelihood that relationships will get worse. Since group members can't control the reactions that others have toward them, they need to do the one thing that they can control, namely, following through on their treatment.

2. *Share your recovery experiences with family members.* This section emphasizes keeping open communications with significant others rather than isolating, avoiding, or attempting to hide symptoms or problems. Improving communications helps to build trust and is likely to elicit support from others when needed.

3. *Include others in your treatment—this may be a relief for both you and others close to you.* Group members frequently find it difficult to ask others for help. Thus, including significant others in the treatment plan and encouraging group members to develop plans for dealing with the early warning signs of relapse are essential. The teaching focus here should include the importance of learning how to ask others for help when appropriate. When discussing this issue, it is useful to ask people what has happened when they previously tried to explain their illnesses to their family members. Many people say that they have a hard time explaining their illnesses to family members, who don't subscribe to the idea that either disorder is in fact an illness. For this reason, encouraging people to use educational resources can be helpful.

4. *Understand that relationships in early recovery often get worse before they get better.* One way of understanding this frequent pattern is to describe the following scenario: A woman who has been clean and sober for only a few days gets a lot of congratulations from AA members and feels quite proud of her 4 days of clean time. Yet her family members remain very upset at all of the difficulties her substance use has caused, and become enraged over the fact that she feels proud of being clean for such a short period of time. Her husband says, "How can you act so proud of yourself just because you haven't behaved like a jerk for 4 whole days, when you've done your best to destroy this family with your addiction for the past 10 years?" The patient reacts to this by saying, "Why should I bother to get sober, when all I get is criticism?"

A key feature of this dynamic is the fact that the substance abuser and her family have very different experiences of recovery, because of several major points:

- *Only the substance abuser knows for sure whether or not he or she is clean and sober.* The suspiciousness and skepticism that family members have may lead them to act in ways that are constantly irritating to the substance abuser. They act that way because they have been frequently disappointed, and they are trying to protect themselves from yet another disappointment.
- *Only the substance abuser knows for sure whether he or she even has any* intention *of remaining clean and sober.* The natural course of SUDs is filled with broken promises, some of which are made sincerely and others that are not. Family members may doubt whether their loved one is truly motivated to stay clean, and even motivated people can relapse.
- *Family members often wait to express their anger until their relative has become sober.* When someone is chronically using drugs and alcohol, attempts to hurt them may not work, because they are so frequently intoxicated that they may not even remember what was said to them. Family members may often "lie in wait" for their relative to become abstinent before they can land a verbal blow.

5. *Try to see things from the other person's point of view.* It helps group members to understand that their situation is not unique, but is shared by others during the process of early recovery. Encourage members to reflect on the difference in their early recovery experience and a family member's early recovery experience, trying to imagine what it might look like from the other side. If they try to see issues from their own point of view as well as that of the other person, then some of these difficulties can be reduced.

With about 8–10 minutes left in the group, you should summarize two or three take-home themes that people should try to remember. You might say something like "Okay, we're near the end of today's group. Let's summarize the main points we discussed today that people should keep in mind." Encourage people to state two or three major concepts from today's session; when this is done, you should say something like "If you only remember two things from today's group, you should remember the following: that the best way to help heal important relationships is by following through on your treatment with the central recovery rule, and by trying to see things from the other person's point of view." You should summarize these main thoughts and write them on the whiteboard, or point them out on the bulletin board and/or the session topic handout. Make sure that everybody understands these main points, then move on to the skill practice assignment.

Step 5: Distribute Handout 4.2 and encourage everyone to pay attention in the upcoming week to opportunities to help repair relationships that need improving (5 minutes).

Tell group members that they should be on the lookout this week for opportunities to "see it from the other side," and not to allow relationship conflicts to interfere with their recovery; they should practice finding ways to defuse these conflicts. If they find this to be difficult during the week, they will have time to ask for help during the next session's review of the skill practice exercises. End the session by saying that you look forward to seeing them again next week.

Dealing with Family Members and Friends

People with bipolar disorder and substance abuse problems commonly experience difficulties in relationships with family members and friends, especially if they live with their family or depend upon family members for many of their day-to-day routines (e.g., transportation, meals, and help with chores and activities). These difficulties may occur for a variety of reasons. First, substance abuse and symptoms of bipolar disorder can be disturbing to people around them. Examples of potentially disturbing symptoms and behaviors include the following (you may wish to highlight any that seem familiar to you and your family):

- **Loss of self-control** (making inappropriate remarks; laughing at inappropriate times; being intoxicated; doing things that frighten others, such as suddenly getting angry or throwing things)
- **Irritability**
- **Being unreliable** (not showing up for family commitments or for work, not taking care of paperwork that places you at risk for losing benefits or housing)
- **Spending too much money** (spending food or rent money on clothes, entertainment, cigarettes, drugs and alcohol, phone charges, lottery tickets, etc.)
- **Having an altered sex drive** (too much sexual desire or loss of sexual desire)
- **Being unpredictable** (e.g., people say to you, "I never can tell what mood you will be in," or "I would like to trust you to mean it this time when you say you won't drink and that you'll take your medication. But you've broken that promise so many times, I don't trust you")

In addition to the problems your behaviors may cause, it is likely that *you* have been disappointed and hurt in relationships as well. One common result of having bipolar disorder and substance abuse is that you and your family members or friends may feel awkward around each other and not know what to say to each other. When people are not sure how to relate to you, they may tend to avoid you. This may make you feel shunned and rejected, and may bring on feelings of resentment that can be a trigger for substance use or for not taking your medication. Examples of thoughts and feelings that can cause problems in relationships are as follows:

- **Depressed thinking.** When you are down on yourself, you believe that everyone else thinks negatively about you; you believe that they view you as worthless, no fun to be with, lazy, or incompetent, and so forth. When you think this way, it shows in your behavior toward others: You will avoid them or feel angry and resentful toward them, and they may not know why you are behaving this way.
- **Manic thinking.** You may have grandiose thoughts about yourself and therefore treat others as if they are unimportant; or you may become paranoid about others, thinking that someone who cares about you really wants to harm you; or you may think unreasonable things (although they seem perfectly reasonable to you, at the time) and then impose these thoughts on others. In most of these cases, people will respond by either getting angry or becoming afraid of you.
- **Relapse thinking.** Rationalizing your desire to use substances generally upsets others, who perceive this to be irresponsible or self-centered thinking.

(cont.)

From *Integrated Group Therapy for Bipolar Disorder and Substance Abuse* by Roger D. Weiss and Hilary Smith Connery. Copyright 2011 by The Guilford Press. Permission to photocopy this material is granted to purchasers of this book for personal use only (see copyright page for details).

WHAT YOU CAN DO TO HELP HEAL WOUNDED RELATIONSHIPS AND STAY ON TRACK WITH YOUR RECOVERY

1. Follow through on your treatment.

The single best way to avoid further problems related to bipolar disorder and substance abuse is to follow through on your treatment. This means that you need to stay drug- and alcohol-free, and to follow through on your psychiatric treatment (medications and other therapy you are prescribed); following the central recovery rule is the key to helping you improve your relationships. If your symptoms are better controlled, and you are clean and sober, others will feel more comfortable with you, and you will also feel more comfortable with them.

2. Share your recovery experiences with family members.

It is sometimes easy to forget to take medications on schedule, or to get to an AA or NA meeting or an appointment with your doctor or clinician. Let your family know that you take these things seriously even if you don't always remember perfectly. Thank your family members for caring about your recovery and for helping you with things like picking up medicine from the pharmacy, packing medication boxes, or driving you to and from a meeting. When you can, share with them things that you learn about controlling your psychiatric symptoms or your urges to drink or use drugs. You may wish to share with them the session handouts or skill practices for this group, so they can see what you are working on and learning.

3. Include others in your treatment—this may be a relief for both you and others close to you.

Your therapist or your doctor can be an excellent source of information for you and your family, to help you understand the symptoms and treatment of bipolar disorder and substance use disorders. Finding a time to discuss these things together with a clinician treating you is a great way to heal misunderstandings and misperceptions about your symptoms and your treatment. People sometimes find that giving relatives the handouts from these groups can be helpful. Ask family members to go to an AA or SMART Recovery meeting to see what that is like, or to attend Al-Anon or Nar-Anon for family support.

4. Understand that relationships in early recovery often get worse before they get better.

People to whom you are close may get very angry at you during periods of mania, depression, or substance use. However, they may not fully show their anger at you until you are sober, when they feel that you are able to listen better. This is precisely at a time when you are feeling good about your early recovery, and their anger may trigger you to feel resentful toward them. It is important to recognize that this can occur, and that it is a temporary step along the path of experiencing recovery with your friends and family. Asking your therapist or doctor to help you to understand what is happening, or to help your family to support your recovery, can be a very effective way of getting everyone through the early recovery stresses.

5. Try to see things from the other person's point of view.

Remember that the other person is not necessarily thinking the way you think. Most arguments and difficulties occur when a person doesn't respect the other person's point of view and make a strong effort to try to understand him or her. You have been through a lot, and so have the people around you; however, you have been through different problems and have different perspectives. Try to understand theirs, and try to help them to understand yours, without fighting, and you will have taken the first step toward healing the relationship.

Skill Practice Homework Sheet:
Dealing with Family Members and Friends

Patient Initials: _____

Date: _____

1. Describe a problem you are having with a family member or a friend that has occurred as the result of symptoms of bipolar disorder.

   _____
   _____
   _____

   What is a positive way that you can deal with this problem?

   _____
   _____
   _____

2. Describe a problem you are having with a family member or a friend that has occurred as the result of your substance abuse problem.

   _____
   _____
   _____

   What is a positive way that you can deal with this problem?

   _____
   _____
   _____

From *Integrated Group Therapy for Bipolar Disorder and Substance Abuse* by Roger D. Weiss and Hilary Smith Connery. Copyright 2011 by The Guilford Press. Permission to photocopy this material is granted to purchasers of this book for personal use only (see copyright page for details).

⟨⟨⟨⟨⟨⟨⟨⟨⟨⟨⟨⟨⟨⟨⟨⟩

Denial, Ambivalence, and Acceptance

SESSION OBJECTIVES

1. Group members will learn that most people with BD and SUDs have mixed feelings about their illnesses and their prescribed treatment, and that their attitude toward treatment may vary during different times in their life.

2. Group members will understand the concepts of denial, ambivalence, and acceptance.

3. Group members will understand how denial, ambivalence, and acceptance can affect behavioral choices.

4. Group members will learn that ambivalence about treatment is common, but acting on this by using substances or stopping treatment for BD (i.e., ignoring the central recovery rule) is very dangerous.

MATERIALS REQUIRED

- Bulletin board with the central recovery rule, routes to recovery or relapse, and Session 5 materials posted.
- Dry erase board and markers.
- Copies of Handout 5.1, "Denial, Ambivalence, and Acceptance."
- Copies of Handout 5.2, "Skill Practice Homework Sheet: Denial, Ambivalence, and Acceptance."

SUMMARY OF SESSION STEPS AND TIME MANAGEMENT

- **Step 1:** Check-in procedure (15 minutes).
- **Step 2:** Review last week's group topic, "Dealing with Family Members and Friends" (2 minutes).
- **Step 3:** Review last week's skill practice questions on Handout 4.2, "Skill Practice Homework Sheet: Dealing with Family Members and Friends" (8 minutes).
- **Step 4:** Distribute Handout 5.1. Explain how denial and ambivalence are a normal part of recovery, and how practicing the central recovery rule despite these thoughts will help to achieve acceptance (30 minutes).
  - Denial is the wish to deny one's illness, its seriousness, and/or the need for treatment.
  - Ambivalence is being unsure about having a problem or needing treatment.
  - Acceptance means that a person knows he or she has an illness and its symptoms can be managed.
  - Denial, ambivalence, and acceptance are on a continuum; group ratings.
  - Acceptance behavior can be practiced even with denial or ambivalent thoughts.
  - Ways to practice acceptance behavior when feeling ambivalent or when in denial.
- **Step 5:** Distribute Handout 5.2 and encourage group members to practice taking good care of themselves in spite of symptoms of denial or ambivalence (5 minutes).

BACKGROUND

The goal of this session is to encourage group members actively to consider the strong association between their attitudes toward recovery and their success in recovery. It is the nature of the illnesses—BD and SUD—that patients will continuously question their diagnoses and wonder whether treatment is really necessary. An obstacle to recovery from SUD and BD is the fact that at various times people either don't believe that they have a problem or don't believe it needs to be taken quite so seriously, or they know in their minds that they have a problem but can't accept it in their hearts. At times they are likely to feel skeptical about the prescribed treatment and to feel burdened and resentful about the need for maintenance treatment. Patients frequently endure phases of treatment during which they think that the treatment itself is worse than the illness being treated.

For example, during episodes of remission, those with BD complain about side effects of medication or may feel that medications interfere with their "creativity" or their "personality." During depressive episodes, patients may perceive that neither medication nor psychotherapy is effective. Many individuals with SUDs "romanticize" the past—especially during the early recovery period (the first several months of abstinence)—and wistfully think back to the time when they were using substances. They may believe that life then was more fun or more interesting, and that being abstinent isn't worth the effort. In addition, you may notice that group members experience contradictory beliefs about BD and substance abuse, sometimes perceiving BD but not substance use to be a problem, or vice versa.

This session informs group members that they may experience changes over time in their attitudes or beliefs about their illnesses and their management, and that monitoring this is essential to prevent acting on these beliefs in a way that will lead to substance use or mood destabilization. This group should give participants the tools they need to cope with changing attitudes toward their treatment without sacrificing their recovery.

Step 1: Check-in procedure (15 minutes).

Following the group leaders' announcements (e.g., expected member or leader absences, changes to the group meeting schedule or site, introductions for new members), all patients should review their weekly progress according to Handout 1.2, "Monitoring Your Symptoms: How to Check In on Your Recovery" (see Session 1). During this time, other group members are discouraged from commenting on the individual's check-in report, since relevant discussions can occur during the review of the skill practice. The group leaders should make brief summary comments that recognize and positively reinforce any thought or behavioral changes that indicate that the group members are making efforts to achieve abstinence and mood stability or to directly apply the central recovery rule. Check-in is also a time for the group leaders to listen carefully for any content that might provide a useful opportunity for the group to discuss this week's group theme; for this session, leaders note on the board any check-in reports that appear to illustrate denial, ambivalence, or acceptance of illness or need for treatment. Good examples include people who share that although they did not feel like coming to group today, they came anyway, knowing that group participation was important to their recovery.

Step 2: Review last week's group topic, "Dealing with Family Members and Friends" (2 minutes).

This step should be shorter than usual to allow more time for Step 3, the review of the skill practice. Ask group members to review briefly the main points of the session: It is common to have difficulty with relationships in early recovery; a person's experience of early recovery is very different from the experience of family members and friends; it is important to try to see things from the other person's perspective; and problems in relationships are never a reason to use substances or to stop treatment for BD. Keep this review brief in order to have more time to review group members' answers to the skill practice.

Step 3: Review last week's skill practice questions on Handout 4.2, "Skill Practice Homework Sheet: Dealing with Family Members and Friends" (8 minutes).

Begin by acknowledging, "This week's skill practice gets into some pretty personal stuff. Who might be brave enough to get us started?" Work hard to elicit support and empathy from group members as they listen to each other's responses. If someone shares a situation that has gone badly, ask group members for suggestions that might help the person better manage the situation. Also note that it is best to avoid certain difficult relationships during early recovery, because the risk for relapse is so great. If this appears to be the situation for a group member, help that member to think about stopping communication or avoiding contact as an early recovery strategy, and to know that it might be better to return to that relationship during a more stable period of recovery.

Step 4: Distribute Handout 5.1. Explain how denial and ambivalence are a normal part of recovery, and how practicing the central recovery rule despite these thoughts will help to achieve acceptance (30 minutes).

Announce today's topic: "Denial, Ambivalence, and Acceptance." Say that this session is designed to help group members think about how their attitudes toward their disorders and their treatment may affect their willingness to stick with treatment. Tell them that it is possible to stick with treatment—and maintain recovery—even when they don't feel like sticking with treatment. This group will help them to learn how to do this.

Next say,

> "Last group we talked about how other people in our lives can affect, sometimes negatively, our commitment to applying the central recovery rule and sticking with treatment. This week we are going to talk about how our *own* shifts in attitude can affect our treatment, and how to stay on track with treatment even when we have mixed feelings about it. Maybe some of you thought about skipping group today, but then decided to show up anyway. That's an example of not allowing a negative thought about treatment to become an action that interferes with treatment, so you probably already have some experience with this."

Denial is the wish to deny one's illness, its seriousness, and/or the need for treatment.

Now say, "I'm sure you have all heard the word *denial* used before to describe a person who doesn't really believe that he or she has a problem with substances, or a problem with mental illness. Maybe some of you have been told before that you are in denial. How would you describe denial?" Allow a few members to respond to this. If a member's check-in report had included some denial, ask members to comment on this. Then, define *denial* as the wish to deny one's illness, its seriousness, or the need for treatment, and write this down on the board. Emphasize that this can occur either with BD or SUD, that it is very common, and that virtually everyone with one or both of these disorders has some degree of denial at times. Also state that denial in the early stages of an illness is a normal, sometimes adaptive reaction, because it takes time for people to accept painful realities. Next, ask group members to suggest some examples of denial (several are listed in session Handout 5.1).

Ambivalence is being unsure about having a problem or needing treatment.

Next, define *ambivalence*:

> "Ambivalence can mean being unsure whether you have a serious problem or need treatment. It can also mean knowing you have a problem but not always wanting to act to make it better. For instance, you might think you have a problem with BD but not

substances, or you might think that if you stopped using substances you would be fine, because you don't believe that you really have BD. Or you may believe that nothing really helps to reduce depression, so why take medications or give up drinking?"

Emphasize the universality of ambivalent feelings about illness and treatment. Stress the idea that all people go through phases of wishing so strongly that things were different that they begin to believe that things actually are not as they appear. Ask group members to share personal experiences of ambivalence and write these on the board.

Acceptance means that a person knows he or she has an illness and its symptoms can be managed.

Then say, "Now we get to acceptance. *Acceptance* means knowing you have an illness and that you can learn to manage its symptoms, so that they do not interfere with the rest of your life."

Denial, ambivalence, and acceptance are on a continuum; group ratings.

Say to group members,

> "Can you see how there is a continuum that begins on one end with denial and ends on the other with acceptance? Probably most people spend most of their time in this wide middle area, with some degree of ambivalence about their illness, although they might at times have a lot of denial and at other times a good deal of acceptance. The idea is that the closer you can get to acceptance, *the easier it is to stay in treatment and to stay well*. When you experience ambivalence about something, you struggle more and feel uncomfortable about it—going back and forth in your thoughts. Acceptance means that the fight in your head is over, so things can just flow more naturally."

Ask group members at this time to rate themselves on a scale from 0 to 10, in which 0 is *complete denial* and 10 is *complete acceptance*; have them rate this separately for BD and for their SUD. Go around the room and ask people for their scores. Most likely, there will be a spread, both within each person (i.e., a person may have greater acceptance of one disorder than the other) and between people (different people may have different levels of acceptance). You might joke with members who rate themselves a "0" that just their acknowledgment of denial moves them closer to acceptance, so they really aren't as far off as they might think.

Acceptance behavior can be practiced even with denial or ambivalent thoughts.

Emphasize that acceptance comes with time, and that it can't be forced on people or made to happen too quickly. Say,

> "This is why we know that people have to 'grow into' the central recovery rule: first you just memorize it, then you begin to be able to use it. Then you learn that it is central to your recovery, so you follow it even when you don't feel like following it. Finally, you follow it because you truly believe in it, and you find that it's not so hard. As they

say in AA, you can "fake it 'til you make it." The reason this strategy works is because there is a big difference between thoughts and attitudes and behavior. You can always choose to do the next right thing even when you think or feel differently from what you are doing."

To illustrate this point, use the analogy of going on a diet to lose weight. Say to the group,

"When you go on a diet, what are the things that you try to avoid eating? (*Allow a few responses.*) Now, are you avoiding these foods because you don't like them anymore? No, of course not! You still really want that chocolate chip cookie, but you don't want the consequence of eating it—weight gain. So you choose to not eat it. People sometimes think that it should be different with giving up drugs and alcohol, that they should no longer *want* to drink or use drugs, but that's unrealistic. What they need to be thinking is 'Of course I want to use! But I know I can't use in safety.' If you're waiting for full acceptance and complete motivation for recovery from bipolar disorder and substance abuse to arrive before you start treatment, you may *never* get into recovery! So you have to work on your recovery even before you feel good about doing it. Don't wait until you *want* to start taking medication or to stop drinking and using drugs before you do it. Knowing that you *have* to do it (even if you don't *want* to) is all that you need to get started. Later, you'll be glad that you did it."

Ways to practice acceptance behavior when feeling ambivalent or when in denial.

At this time, ask the group, "What would you do if you noticed yourself moving toward denial?" The group members are taught that they first need to be able to identify symptoms of denial and ambivalence, then to respond to these symptoms with recovery behaviors. Key recovery behaviors include talking to someone else about their thoughts or feelings and sticking with the central recovery rule. Ask members to identify good people to talk to and write a list on the board that includes their doctors, therapists, family members, sponsors, or trusted friends. Tell people that denial tends to grow when they don't get feedback from other people, and that people with substance abuse problems and mental illness typically have "blind spots," which means that they cannot always see the whole picture. Sometimes SUDs and BD (particularly mania) are called "diseases of denial," because one symptom may be that people with these disorders don't feel ill. They therefore need to include someone else's observations or opinions to help them to have a fuller perspective.

With about 8–10 minutes left in the group, summarize two or three take-home themes that people should try to remember. You might say something like "Okay, we're near the end of today's group. Let's summarize the main points we discussed today that people should keep in mind." Encourage people to state two or three major concepts from today's session; when this is done, you should say something like

"If you only remember a few things from today's group, you should remember the following: that feeling ambivalent about recovery is common and natural, particularly in the early stages of recovery. However, acting on this ambivalence by using substances or stopping bipolar disorder treatment is very dangerous; the way to deal with ambivalent thoughts or denial thoughts is to follow the central recovery rule, and this will help you to achieve acceptance."

You should summarize these main thoughts and write them on the whiteboard, or point them out on the bulletin board and/or the session topic handout. Make sure that everybody understands these main points, then move on to the skill practice assignment.

Step 5: Distribute Handout 5.2 and encourage group members to practice taking good care of themselves in spite of symptoms of denial or ambivalence (5 minutes).

Ask group members to pay attention this week to symptoms of denial or ambivalence, and to practice talking with someone they trust about their thoughts and feelings. Remind them that they can "fake it 'til they make it" by applying the central recovery rule. End the session by saying that you look forward to seeing them all next week.

Denial, Ambivalence, and Acceptance

WHAT IS DENIAL?

Denial is the wish to deny the existence or seriousness of one's illness and/or the need for treatment. Denial can occur with either BD or SUD, and is a common experience in recovery. Almost everyone with one or both of these disorders has some **denial thoughts** at times; but if these thoughts lead to **denial behaviors** (e.g., not taking medication, or using drugs or alcohol), then a person enters very dangerous situations that threaten recovery.

HOW CAN YOU RECOGNIZE DENIAL?

Denial can appear in your *thoughts*, your *behavior*, or both.

Examples of denial thoughts:

- Believing that **just** one drink or **just** one line of cocaine or **just** one joint won't do any harm.
- Believing that medications you have been prescribed (lithium, valproate, risperidone, olanzapine, etc.) aren't helpful, that you would feel better without them, and that you should stop them on your own.

Examples of denial behaviors:

- Using drugs or alcohol because you believe they won't do any harm.
- Not taking your medications as prescribed because you believe you don't need them.
- Not going to a therapy appointment because you believe you don't need it.

What to do when you notice yourself having denial thoughts:

Talk to someone else: your doctor, your therapist, a family member, your sponsor, or a trusted friend. Denial tends to grow when you don't get feedback from other people. Remember that people with alcohol or drug problems typically have "blind spots": parts of themselves that they cannot see. Because of this, they need someone else to help them look at their behavior. When you start having denial thoughts, you're heading for trouble! Don't give in to them! **Remember the central recovery rule: " No matter what, don't drink, don't use drugs, and take your medication as prescribed—NO MATTER WHAT!"** When you start doubting this rule, you need to talk to someone!

WHAT IS AMBIVALENCE?

Ambivalence means being unsure whether you have a serious problem, or whether you need treatment. Sometimes you think that you do, and other times, you think that you don't. Like denial, ambivalence is very common. Almost everyone has ambivalence at various times; sometimes it is stronger than at other times. How can you recognize ambivalence?

Examples of ambivalence thoughts:

- Wondering whether you really have bipolar disorder, or wondering whether your drug or alcohol problem is really as serious as other people think.
- Wondering whether your medication is doing anything besides causing side effects, and thinking that you might experiment with stopping your medication on your own.

(cont.)

From *Integrated Group Therapy for Bipolar Disorder and Substance Abuse* by Roger D. Weiss and Hilary Smith Connery. Copyright 2011 by The Guilford Press. Permission to photocopy this material is granted to purchasers of this book for personal use only (see copyright page for details).

Examples of ambivalence behaviors:

- Taking medication irregularly or attending treatment or self-help groups irregularly, based on changing your mind about how serious your problem is.
- "Running out" of medication: calling your doctor for a refill only *after* you have run out, so that you miss doses.
- Telling your doctor, therapist, family, and sponsor that you don't want to drink or use drugs, then hanging around with people who you know will be drinking and using drugs in front of you, and inviting you to use with them.

What to do when you are having ambivalent thoughts:

As with denial, it is important to continue to talk to other people when you feel ambivalent about sobriety or treatment, and not to act on those thoughts or feelings. Even if you don't **feel** like staying in treatment, stay in treatment, **no matter what**! Even if you **feel** like drinking or using drugs, don't do it, **no matter what**! Talking to other people who have coped successfully with these illnesses is particularly helpful during these times. By talking to these people, you can realize that it is possible to enjoy life despite these illnesses, and you can find out how **other** people have done so. This type of information can help motivate you to continue working hard at your recovery, even when you get discouraged and are tempted to give up. You'll be glad later.

WHAT IS ACCEPTANCE?

Acceptance means understanding (1) that you have these two illnesses, combined as "bipolar substance abuse"; (2) that you need to treat this combined disorder; (3) that you need to **continue** to treat it; and (4) that **that's okay**. Acceptance gives you peace of mind. Although the process of arriving at acceptance is difficult, getting there and doing your best to stay there is worth the effort.

Examples of acceptance thoughts:

- Not feeling deprived, but instead feeling good about being drug- and alcohol-free.
- Being grateful that you have found a medication that reduces unwanted symptoms of your bipolar disorder.

Examples of acceptance behaviors:

- Doing what you need to do in your treatment of substance abuse and bipolar disorder without feeling resentful, even if medication causes some side effects.
- Making sure that you remember to take your medication with you if you go away for the weekend, and that you have enough medication to last until you return home.

What to do when you believe that you are accepting your illnesses:

Congratulations! Remember, however, that once you have begun accepting your illnesses, you have to keep working at it, or you may shift back into ambivalence, or even into denial. Always remain watchful for these other thought or behavior patterns, so that you can take the appropriate steps to keep up and strengthen your acceptance.

Skill Practice Homework Sheet: Denial, Ambivalence, and Acceptance

Patient Initials: _____

Date: _____

List below a symptom of denial of substance abuse that you have had, what you have done about it in the past that has been helpful, what else you will do about it in the coming week, and what person you will talk to if you notice denial thoughts again. After you have done this, please do the same exercise for bipolar disorder. If you have trouble thinking of an example, you may wish to ask a family member or friend to remind you of a time when you showed denial about your illnesses.

Substance Abuse

1. List a symptom of denial of your substance abuse.

   _____

   _____

   _____

2. What have you done in the past to successfully overcome this symptom?

   _____

   _____

   _____

3. What else will you do this week to overcome this symptom?

   _____

   _____

   _____

4. Whom will you talk to if you notice denial thoughts happening again?

   _____

   _____

   _____

(cont.)

From *Integrated Group Therapy for Bipolar Disorder and Substance Abuse* by Roger D. Weiss and Hilary Smith Connery. Copyright 2011 by The Guilford Press. Permission to photocopy this material is granted to purchasers of this book for personal use only (see copyright page for details).

Bipolar Disorder

1. List a symptom of denial of your bipolar disorder.

    _____

    _____

    _____

2. What have you done in the past to successfully overcome this symptom?

    _____

    _____

    _____

3. What else will you do this week to overcome this symptom?

    _____

    _____

    _____

4. Whom will you talk to if you notice denial thoughts happening again?

    _____

    _____

    _____

◯◯◯◯◯◯◯◯◯◯◯◯◯◯◯◯◯◯◯

Reading Your Signals

Recognizing Early Warning Signs of Trouble

SESSION OBJECTIVES

1. Group members will learn that before they become manic or depressed, there are often telltale signs and symptoms warning them that they are entering a mood episode. They will be able to define these symptoms (changes in sleep, energy, appetite, libido, and thought content and speed).

2. Group members will learn that before they relapse to using substances, there are often telltale signs and symptoms warning them that they are at risk for relapse. They will be able to define these symptoms and the acronym "BUDDing."

3. Group members will learn how to practice daily symptom monitoring to detect warning signs of recurrence and relapse.

4. Group members will know what to do if they believe they are at risk for recurrence or relapse (practice the central recovery rule and alert their treatment team right away).

MATERIALS REQUIRED

- Bulletin board with the central recovery rule, routes to recovery or relapse, and Session 6 materials posted.
- Dry erase board and markers.
- Copies of Handout 6.1, "Reading Your Signals: Recognizing Early Warning Signs of Trouble."
- Copies of Handout 6.2, "Skill Practice Homework Sheet: Reading Your Signals: Recognizing Early Warning Signs of Trouble."

SUMMARY OF SESSION STEPS AND TIME MANAGEMENT

- **Step 1:** Check-in procedure (15 minutes).
- **Step 2:** Review last week's group topic, "Denial, Ambivalence, and Acceptance" (5 minutes).
- **Step 3:** Review last week's skill practice questions on Handout 5.2, "Skill Practice Homework Sheet: Denial, Ambivalence, and Acceptance" (5 minutes).
- **Step 4:** Distribute Handout 6.1. Introduce the idea of looking for and responding to early warning signs of a mood episode or substance use relapse (30 minutes).
  - Determining the earliest symptoms of mood episodes or substance use relapse.
  - Introduce daily symptom monitoring.
  - Building Up to Drinking and Drugging (BUDDing).
  - Other people can help with recognizing early symptoms.
  - Top 10 strategies for dealing with early symptoms.
- **Step 5:** Distribute Handout 6.2. Review the skill practice for the next group; ask members to keep a daily symptom-monitoring log (5 minutes).

BACKGROUND

This group session teaches patients to actively monitor their symptoms of bipolar disorder and substance use disorder for the purpose of recognizing early warning signs of entering a mood episode or a substance use relapse. The goal is to empower group members who otherwise would experience mood episode recurrence or substance use relapse episodes as beyond their control. This perceived loss of control is one of the most painful symptoms of these disorders; here, the group leaders will teach group members that they have the ability to watch for early symptoms and to respond to them quickly to prevent relapse and recurrence—to gain more control of their illnesses rather than having their illnesses control them.

This session also introduces group members to *daily symptom monitoring*, a simple system for rating their illness symptoms every day on a scale of 0–10, in which a score of 0 represents being *symptom-free*, and 10 indicates *the worst symptoms ever experienced*. Members are taught to recognize early signs and symptoms of mood destabilization or the approach of relapse to substance use. Group leaders review early symptoms listed in session Handout 6.1 and emphasize that some warning signs are common to most people (e.g., having increased desire to use substances, or noticing increased anxiety) while others may be specific to a particular person's pattern of substance use relapse or mood episode recurrence (e.g., desire to use substances only when in contact with a specific person, or becoming mentally preoccupied with one topic of individual interest, such as the origin of the earth). Members will practice rating their current symptoms for BD and for SUD, and will review the strategies outlined in Handout 6.1 for responding to early warning signs.

Step 1: Check-in procedure (15 minutes).

Following the group leaders' announcements (e.g., expected member or leader absences, changes to the group meeting schedule or site, introductions for new members), all patients should review their weekly progress according to Handout 1.2, "Monitoring Your Symptoms: How to Check In on Your Recovery" (see Session 1). During this time, other group members are discouraged from commenting on the individual's check-in report, since relevant discussions can occur during the review of the skill practice. The group leaders should make brief summary comments that recognize and positively reinforce any thought or behavioral changes that indicate that the group members are making efforts to achieve abstinence and mood stability or to directly apply the central recovery rule. Check-in is also a time for the group leaders to listen carefully for any content that might provide a useful opportunity for the group to discuss this week's group theme; for this session, leaders will note on the board any check-in reports that include substance use, or symptoms of depression or mania.

Step 2: Review last week's group topic, "Denial, Ambivalence, and Acceptance" (5 minutes).

Ask group members to briefly review the definitions for each of these terms, and to provide an example of each as a thought and as a behavior. Ask them to predict what could happen if they acted on these thoughts and behaviors instead of following the central recovery rule.

Step 3: Review last week's skill practice questions on Handout 5.2, "Skill Practice Homework Sheet: Denial, Ambivalence, and Acceptance" (5 minutes).

Use this exercise to highlight any evidence that members are working toward acceptance of their illnesses and treatment; give positive reinforcement for this. For members who are struggling with denial and ambivalence, enlist the rest of the group to come up with ideas that may help that individual to move closer to acceptance.

Step 4: Distribute Handout 6.1. Introduce the idea of looking for and responding to early warning signs of a mood episode or substance use relapse (30 minutes).

Determining the earliest symptoms of mood episodes or substance use relapse.

Announce today's topic: "Reading Your Signals: Recognizing Early Warning Signs of Trouble." Say that this session will emphasize that it is possible to halt the progression of a mood episode recurrence or a substance use relapse; this session is intended to teach group members how to recognize early trouble and to stop it before it becomes a full-blown problem.

Begin by asking the group, "How can you tell if you are getting depressed or manic, or are about to start using substances? What are some of your earliest symptoms?" Write down responses in three columns (depression, mania, and substance use) to organize these early signs of trouble. Use the examples in Handout 6.1 to supplement this discussion.

If people report mood symptoms during the check-in, guide them through the process of identifying their earliest warning signs of a mood episode—including thoughts, behaviors, and physical symptoms or changes that are noticeable (sleeping more or less, eating more or less, feeling tired or more energetic, thinking quickly or having difficulty thinking, feeling increased or decreased sex drive). Point out that some symptoms are experienced nearly universally as early warning signs, and others are specific to particular individuals, but all are patterns that a person can learn to recognize as signaling trouble ahead.

Introduce daily symptom monitoring.

Next, introduce group members to *daily symptom monitoring*. Explain that they can keep a record or chart of their symptom ratings (and other early warning signs, such as the number of hours of sleep) on a calendar for the purpose of identifying and heading off a mood episode or substance use relapse. Explain the 0 to 10-point rating scale, in which 0 is *no symptoms at all* and 10 is *the worst symptoms I've ever had.* Tell them that you are going to practice this rating in group today, with one rating for mood symptoms and another for the substance abuse symptoms. Then go around the room and ask group members to rate their symptoms. Ask them to identify which symptoms led them to give that rating. Ask members with ratings of 5 or higher if they would have rated this differently last week, and if so, what has changed. This can help to demonstrate how an individual can monitor the progression of symptoms leading up to a mood episode or a relapse.

Building Up to Drinking and Drugging (BUDDing).

Next, write the word *BUDDing* on the board and ask whether any group members have heard this term used before. If so, ask them what they understand it to mean. Define BUDDing as Building Up to Drinking and Drugging. Review the symptoms of BUDDing listed in session Handout 6.1 (argumentativeness, not listening to others, not taking treatment as seriously as before, and feeling overly confident), and ask members if they can recall a time when they were BUDDing and then relapsed to substance use soon afterward.

Other people can help with recognizing early symptoms.

Ask members if they failed to listen to other people who warned them that they were heading for trouble; if so, ask what were their reasons for ignoring these warnings. Remind people that both SUD and BD are characterized by "blind spots" (sometimes known as *denial*), and that everyone needs other people to help them to see their blind spots. Say to the group, "If you get advice from people and immediately dismiss it, you are probably going to get into trouble. You can disagree with other people who tell you that you are heading for trouble, but if you don't think very hard about what they are saying and appreciate the advice, you are not making use of an important tool available to you for staying in control of your illnesses."

Top 10 strategies for dealing with early symptoms.

Finally, review the "top 10" strategies on Handout 6.1 for what to do if you recognize early signs of a mood episode or substance use relapse. These strategies are as follows:

1. *Call your therapist, doctor, or nurse.* It is possible that talking about what's going on and/or changing your medication or your dose may help to avoid symptoms getting out of control.
2. *Don't stay in bed.* Get up and try to do some of your usual routine. If you find that you can't, ask someone you trust (sponsor, family) for help.
3. *Avoid isolating yourself.* Get outside, go somewhere with other people you trust.
4. *Distract yourself.* Stay busy and focus on something other than your symptoms. Negative thoughts often decrease if you concentrate on doing something productive, like working or running an errand.
5. *Avoid overstimulating situations* that can make anxiety and disturbing thoughts worse.
6. *Try to maintain a regular sleep pattern of at least 7 hours per day.* If you need some medication to help you to get to sleep or to stay asleep, ask your doctor or nurse for help.
7. *Attend an AA, NA, SMART Recovery, or Dual Recovery Anonymous meeting and ask for help.*
8. *Call your AA or NA sponsor* and tell him or her that you are in a high-risk situation, and are asking for help.
9. *Stay away from people who tempt you to use substances or who tend to upset you emotionally.*
10. *Exercise or meditate* to relieve stress and to improve your sense of well-being.
    And, of course, don't forget the central recovery rule!

Invite group members to suggest other strategies, if they have found something that works well for them. Emphasize that other people can also help them monitor their recovery, since sometimes others will notice changes in mood or behavior that the individual does not notice. Emphasize that being open-minded about this kind of feedback from others will help their recovery.

With about 8–10 minutes to go in the group, you should summarize two or three take-home themes that people should try to remember. You might say something like "Okay, we're near the end of today's group. Let's summarize the main points we discussed today that people should keep in mind." Encourage people to state a couple of main points; when this is done, you should say something like "If you only remember two things from today's group, you should remember the following: Monitor yourselves carefully for early warning signs of a mood episode or substance use relapse, and seek help from others, if they notice these early warning signs, rather than isolating yourself." You should summarize these main thoughts and write them on the whiteboard, or point them out on the bulletin board and/or the session topic handout. Make sure that everybody understands these main points, then move on to the skill practice assignment.

Step 5: Distribute Handout 6.2. Review the skill practice for the next group; ask members to keep a daily symptom-monitoring log (5 minutes).

Ask group members to keep a calendar for every day in the upcoming week, in which they record their symptom ratings; they should bring their calendars to next week's session. Tell them that this small daily effort can pay off in huge ways if they use it to avoid another mood or substance use episode. End the session by saying that you look forward to seeing them all next week.

Reading Your Signals: Recognizing Early Warning Signs of Trouble

One of the most important things you can do for your recovery is to pay careful attention to early warning signs of relapse to substance use or a return of bipolar disorder symptoms. In Session 1 ("It's Two against One, but You Can Win!"), we reviewed the general symptoms of substance use disorders and bipolar disorder. In this session, we emphasize the importance of getting to know your own symptom pattern, since everyone experiences different symptoms at different times. Once you know your own early warning signs, you may be able to head off a substance use relapse or a serious mood episode, and spare yourself and those around you a great deal of pain. Don't expect this to come easily; it won't. You need to pay attention every day by monitoring changes in your moods, your thoughts, your physical symptoms, and your urges to use substances in order to know whether you're heading for trouble.

MONITORING YOUR MOOD SYMPTOMS AND YOUR DESIRE FOR SUBSTANCE USE

A simple way to get started with monitoring your mood symptoms and your desire to use substances is to keep a monitoring chart every day. It doesn't have to be complicated, and it can be done in a matter of seconds. An example includes monitoring the typical symptoms you have had in the past when your bipolar disorder or substance use was uncontrolled. Use a scale of 0–10 every day; a score of 0 means *no symptoms at all*, and a score of 10 means *the worst symptoms you have ever had*. Give yourself two separate ratings: one for mood symptoms and another for substance abuse. (You can be stable in one but not in the other, stable in both, or unstable in both.) Doing this every day will help you to get a sense of how you're doing over a period of time. You will therefore be able to tell whether things are improving, getting worse, or staying the same.

EARLY WARNING SIGNS OF SUBSTANCE ABUSE

The earliest warning signs for substance abuse usually involve thoughts that indicate **relapse thinking**. Examples of this are as follows:

- "My substance abuse problem isn't so bad."
- "My problem was with cocaine, not with alcohol or marijuana."
- "I know that having a drink is a bad idea, but I just need some relief, to self-medicate."

The three major patterns of relapse thinking are as follows:

1. **Minimizing the problems** associated with your substance use
   - "I can control it. It wasn't so bad."
2. **Thinking positively about your substance use**
   - "I'm less anxious and depressed when I use."
3. **Not caring about the negative consequences**
   - "I just need some relief tonight; I don't care what happens tomorrow."

When you find yourself thinking in any of these ways, you're in trouble!

(cont.)

From *Integrated Group Therapy for Bipolar Disorder and Substance Abuse* by Roger D. Weiss and Hilary Smith Connery. Copyright 2011 by The Guilford Press. Permission to photocopy this material is granted to purchasers of this book for personal use only (see copyright page for details).

A second sign of trouble involves **relapse behavior**. This usually follows relapse thinking, but you may recognize relapse behavior without having recognized the relapse thinking beforehand. **Relapse behavior typically involves entering high-risk situations**: going to bars, seeing people that you used to use substances with, hanging around in places that remind you of drug or alcohol use.

Even if you have relapse thinking or relapse behavior, you still do not have to use substances. Remember your coping skills, which are described in greater detail in the session entitled "Identifying and Fighting Triggers," including the **AAA method** of dealing with internal or external triggers to use (**avoid** triggers, avoid facing triggers **alone**, when you are triggered distract yourself with **activities** or get **away**).

EARLY WARNING SIGNS OF MOOD EPISODES

Early warning signs of mood episodes may vary for different people, but often include the following:

- Irritability
- Sleep problems (either too much or too little)
- Worrying that others are talking about you, following you, planning to hurt you
- Feeling unsafe
- Crying without knowing why you're crying
- Feeling that you want to be left alone
- Forgetting to eat or to take a shower, or feeling that everyday activities take too much effort
- People who know you comment that you are "acting strangely" or keep asking you, "What's wrong?"
- You can't think clearly or your mind either stays on one thought all the time or jumps around from thought to thought

LISTENING TO OTHERS:
ANOTHER METHOD TO CATCH EARLY WARNING SIGNS OF TROUBLE

A second and very important way of learning about early warning signs is to hear about them from other people. For substance use, the term **BUDDing** may be used; this stands for **B**uilding **U**p to **D**rinking and **D**rugging. Signs of BUDDing include the following:

- Argumentativeness
- Not listening to others
- Not taking one's treatment as seriously as before
- Feeling overly confident

This may occur in the presence or in the absence of actual desire to use substances. If you get advice from people and immediately dismiss it, you are probably heading for trouble. You can disagree with other people who tell you that you are heading for trouble, but if you don't think hard about what people are saying and appreciate the advice, you are likely to get into trouble.

(cont.)

"TOP 10" THINGS YOU CAN DO IF YOU RECOGNIZE
EARLY WARNING SIGNS OF TROUBLE

1. **Call your therapist, doctor, or nurse**. It is possible that talking about what's going on and/or changing your medication or your dose may help to avoid symptoms getting out of control.

2. **Don't stay in bed**. Get up and try to do some of your usual routine. If you find that you can't, ask someone you trust for help (sponsor, family).

3. **Avoid isolating yourself**. Get outside; go somewhere with other people you trust.

4. **Distract yourself**. Stay busy and focus on something other than your symptoms. Negative thoughts often decrease if you concentrate on doing something productive, like working or running an errand.

5. **Avoid overstimulating situations** that can make anxiety and disturbing thoughts worse.

6. **Try to maintain a regular sleep pattern of at least 7 hours per day**. If you need some medication to help you to get to sleep or to stay asleep, ask your doctor or nurse for help.

7. **Attend an AA, NA, SMART Recovery, or Dual Recovery Anonymous meeting and ask for help**.

8. **Call your AA or NA sponsor** and tell him or her that you are in a high-risk situation, and are asking for help.

9. **Stay away from people who tempt you to use substances, or who tend to upset you emotionally**.

10. **Exercise or meditate** to relieve stress and to improve your sense of well-being.

And, of course, don't forget the central recovery rule!

Skill Practice Homework Sheet: Reading Your Signals: Recognizing Early Warning Signs of Trouble

Patient Initials: _____

Date: _____

1. List one of your early warning signs for bipolar disorder.

    _____

    _____

2. List one thing that you can do about this to keep your mood symptoms controlled.

    _____

    _____

3. Name at least one person you would trust to help you if you noticed that you were having increased mood symptoms.

    _____

    _____

4. Name at least one person you would listen to if that person expressed concern that you were showing increased mood symptoms.

    _____

    _____

5. List one of your early warning signs for substance abuse.

    _____

    _____

6. List one thing that you can do about this to help avoid using drugs or alcohol.

    _____

    _____

7. Name at least one person you would be able to talk to if you noticed that you were having increased urges to use alcohol or drugs.

    _____

    _____

8. Name at least one person you would listen to if that person expressed concern that you were showing signs of "BUDDing."

    _____

    _____

From *Integrated Group Therapy for Bipolar Disorder and Substance Abuse* by Roger D. Weiss and Hilary Smith Connery. Copyright 2011 by The Guilford Press. Permission to photocopy this material is granted to purchasers of this book for personal use only (see copyright page for details).

Refusing Alcohol and Drugs

Thinking It Through and Knowing What to Say

SESSION OBJECTIVES

1. Group members will learn that staying away from high-risk situations is the best way to avoid substance use, and that turning down an offer to use substances is extremely difficult to do, especially in early recovery.

2. Group members will learn a technique called "snapshot versus video thinking" to help them think through their decisions about refusing alcohol and drugs in a way that will facilitate recovery.

3. Group members will develop their own strategies for turning down an offer to use.

4. Group members will practice executing these substance refusal skills, role-playing challenging situations with other group members.

MATERIALS REQUIRED

- Bulletin board with the central recovery rule, routes to recovery or relapse, and Session 7 materials posted.

- Dry erase board and markers.

- Copies of Handout 7.1, "Refusing Alcohol and Drugs: Thinking It Through and Knowing What to Say."

- Copies of Handout 7.2, "Skill Practice Homework Sheet: Refusing Alcohol and Drugs: Thinking It Through and Knowing What to Say."

SUMMARY OF SESSION STEPS AND TIME MANAGEMENT

- **Step 1:** Check-in procedure (15 minutes).
- **Step 2:** Review last week's group topic, "Reading Your Signals: Recognizing Early Warning Signs of Trouble" (5 minutes).
- **Step 3:** Review last week's skill practice questions on Handout 6.2, "Skill Practice Homework Sheet: Reading Your Signals: Recognizing Early Warning Signs of Trouble" (5 minutes).
- **Step 4:** Distribute Handout 7.1, and discuss (1) avoidance of high-risk situations and (2) skills to refuse drugs or alcohol if offered (30 minutes).
  - Review the "AAA method" for fighting triggers.
  - Discuss group experiences of refusing or not refusing drug and alcohol offers.
  - Group members learn "snapshot versus video thinking" and brainstorm refusal strategies; they discuss how to strengthen their responses.
  - Group members role-play drug or alcohol refusal.
- **Step 5:** Distribute Handout 7.2. Review the skill practice for the next group, and ask all members to keep developing and practicing their refusal skills this week (5 minutes).

BACKGROUND

This group session reminds members that, whenever possible, they should avoid entering situations in which someone may offer them alcohol or drugs, since the immediate availability of alcohol and drugs greatly increases urges to use and thus increases their risk of substance use. Sometimes, however, an individual can be caught off guard by a high-risk situation. Mention that this is much harder to manage than responding to early warning signals. In this case, the best thing to do is to leave the situation immediately. If that is not possible, though, one needs to be prepared with substance refusal skills.

Most members will report a history of failure to refuse a substance that is offered to them. Point out that this is expected, because the greatest risk for relapse is having immediate access to the substance of choice. These skills are often extremely difficult to apply in real situations, and should be considered a *last* line of defense. Being prepared for substance refusal means developing a strategy for (1) *deciding* to say "no," then (2) developing a strategy for *saying* "no," then (3) *rehearsing* these refusal responses until they become automatic. Tell group members that rehearsing drink and drug refusal skills may save them from relapsing in unexpected emergency situations, but this will have a much greater chance of being effective only if they have practiced these skills so thoroughly that they become automatic responses to these high-risk situations. Members will spend time in group role playing difficult situations, in which one member invites another to use substances, and that member has to refuse the offer. In this way, group members provide each other feedback on how effectively they executed their drink and drug refusal and together develop improved personal strategies for refusing offers to use substances.

Step 1: Check-in procedure (15 minutes).

Following the group leaders' announcements (e.g., expected member or leader absences, changes to the group meeting schedule or site, introductions for new members), all patients should review their weekly progress according to Handout 1.2, "Monitoring Your Symptoms: How to Check In on Your Recovery" (see Session 1). During this time, other group members are discouraged from commenting on the individual's check-in report, since relevant discussions can occur during the review of the skill practice. The group leaders should make brief summary comments that recognize and positively reinforce any thought or behavioral changes that indicate that the group members are making efforts to achieve abstinence and mood stability or to directly apply the central recovery rule. Check-in is also a time for group leaders to listen carefully for any content that might provide a useful opportunity for the group to discuss this week's group theme; for this session, leaders will note any reports of high-risk situations in which alcohol or drugs were available to group members.

Step 2: Review last week's group topic, "Reading Your Signals: Recognizing Early Warning Signs of Trouble" (5 minutes).

Ask group members to list common early warning signs for depression, mania, and substance use relapse. Invite members who remembered to bring in their daily symptom monitoring calendar to share what they observed about their symptoms of BD and SUD, and ask them if they found this helpful. Ask any member with a symptom rating of 5 or greater to think back to the preceding week and to estimate whether their symptoms were any better 2 weeks ago. If the answer is "yes," help them to consider what early warning signs they might have picked up on back then, and what they might have done then to prevent their symptoms from progressing this week. If they have difficulty with this exercise, invite other group members to consider their situation and to suggest recovery behaviors or skills appropriate to those situations.

Step 3: Review last week's skill practice questions on Handout 6.2, "Skill Practice Homework Sheet: Reading Your Signals: Recognizing Early Warning Signs of Trouble" (5 minutes).

Make a point to positively reinforce any evidence that members are being open-minded and receptive to other people's feedback about their symptoms.

Step 4: Distribute Handout 7.1, and discuss (1) avoidance of high-risk situations and (2) skills to refuse drugs or alcohol if offered (30 minutes).

Review the "AAA method" for fighting triggers.

Announce today's topic: "Refusing Alcohol and Drugs: Thinking It Through and Knowing What to Say." Tell the group that even though it is *always* safer to avoid high-risk situations and people, sometimes you cannot do so. Say that in these instances, it is possible to refuse an offer to drink or to use drugs—but only if they are highly prepared to do so. Say to the group that this session will help members to prepare to refuse such an offer.

Then say, "Even though our main goal today is to develop and practice drink and drug refusal skills, let's first review what you learned in Session 2, 'Identifying and Fighting Triggers.' Does anyone remember what the *A*'s stand for in the 'AAA method' of fighting triggers to use?" Write the correct answers on the board (*Avoid* triggers when possible. Don't face triggers *alone*. Distract yourself from triggers by getting *active* or getting *away*). Make the point that in the last of these situations, getting away may require telling a person that you do not intend to drink or to use drugs; being able to pull this off successfully requires a well-rehearsed plan for how to tell someone this.

Discuss group experiences of refusing or not refusing drug or alcohol offers.

Ask members to talk about a time they have been able to refuse successfully an offer to drink or use drugs; ask what they think made it possible for them to succeed. Write examples on the board. Then, ask if anyone tried to do this but failed and ended up using; write these examples on the board as well, in another column. See whether group members can identify why one person's efforts failed while another's succeeded. Ask if anyone can suggest a change to the failed strategy that might have resulted in success. Try to get as many members talking about this as possible, so you can demonstrate that members have problem-solving skills and can develop improved self-efficacy if they think about a situation *before* getting there.

Group members learn "snapshot versus video thinking" and brainstorm refusal strategies; they discuss how to strengthen their responses.

Ask people to think about how they would say "no" to someone offering them alcohol or drugs. While they are thinking of this, and before the role plays, you can say,

> "The first thing to bear in mind when someone offers you drugs or alcohol is that you are dealing with two issues: *whether* to say no, then *how* to say no. The first decision can be difficult, because being around drugs and alcohol will increase your desire for them. So you need to develop a strategy to help you make a good decision in this situation. A key factor in determining whether you move toward recovery or relapse is the type of decisions you make. These decisions come up often: 'Should I go to this party or stay home?'; 'Should I have a drink or not?'; 'Should I take my medication as prescribed or not?'"

Tell them one strategy that will help them make a good decision for their recovery is *thinking through the decision*. Say that they have likely heard the term "think through the drink." What exactly does that mean, and how can they know whether they *are* or *are not* thinking it through? Many times, people make decisions they regret. They later realize that they had not thought it through, although they believed at the time that they *were* thinking it through. How can people tell at the time whether they are thinking through a decision or not? Tell them that the technique called "snapshot versus video thinking" may help them to figure this out.

Tell them that a common example of *not* thinking through a decision is imagining only the *short-term* consequences of the decision. You can say,

"For example, if you feel depressed and are thinking about drinking as a way to relieve your depression, one way to *not* think through that decision is just to think about how you will feel after having your first drink. When you think about that, you may imagine that you will feel less depressed. In this case, you are only thinking about a very short period of time: the feeling that you will have after one drink. In other words, you are taking a "snapshot" of how you will feel after a single drink, and are focusing on that brief moment as the result of your drinking.

"Thinking it through involves imagining a *video* rather than a *snapshot*. Imagine that your drinking will produce a long video, not a snapshot. Tell yourself to 'watch the whole video' and see how you will feel after *four* drinks or *eight* drinks. How will you feel tomorrow? How about the next day? How about the day after that? Imagine how you will feel if you go on a binge. Even though one drink may temporarily improve your mood, most people find that their depression the next day, after a drinking binge, is worse than it was before they started drinking. Imagine how other people might respond. Imagine the increased desire you will have to keep drinking if you start with 'a drink' tonight. Imagine having to reset your sobriety date. Continue to say to yourself, 'And then what? An then what? And then what?' In other words, imagine watching a long video of *all* of the consequences of 'a drink.' That is what *thinking it through* really means: using *video thinking* instead of *snapshot thinking*."

Tell that them that thinking through decisions is equally relevant when dealing with taking medication. Stopping medication because of side effects may help people to feel better temporarily, but that is just a "snapshot"—the *short-term* consequence. Group members should be encouraged instead to "watch the whole video," which would include an increased likelihood of depression or mania. Similarly, people may think that stopping medication could make them hypomanic; they might recall their manic episodes fondly, particularly in the early stages of hypomania, when they felt terrific. That is another example of *snapshot thinking*, however. When thinking about mania, they should again "watch the whole video"—spending sprees that lead to huge debt problems and the crashing depression that follows the manic episode. Thinking through the decision by "watching the whole video" can help to improve the quality of group members' decisions, thus helping their recovery.

Now say, "So let's assume now that you have *decided* to say 'no.' That's a big step, but now you have to figure out *how* to do it. In your session handouts, there are "Five Rules to Help You Say No."

Write down the following *five rules for formulating a strong response:*

1. *Don't lie.* This will make you nervous and less certain of your response.
2. You don't have to tell everyone, "I'm a recovering alcoholic/addict."
3. You can say different things in different situations, as long as what you say is true.
4. Don't get upset if someone asks you to drink or use drugs; just refuse calmly.
5. Say something that you are comfortable saying.

Ask members to think about these rules, and to make sure that their responses follow these general rules.

Group members role-play drug or alcohol refusal.

Ask two people to volunteer as the "offerer" and the "refuser," and provide realistic situations that members might encounter. Direct the offerer to persist a bit in a way that might happen in real life, such as asking why a person doesn't want a drink. At the end of each role play, ask the refuser, "How did that go for you? Do you think that it would have worked? Why or why not? Is there a way in which you would change your answer now?" Also ask other group members to rate the refuser on the strength of the refusal, and to offer suggestions for improvement. At the end of this session, answer any questions members may still have about how to refuse a drink or drug. Some members may believe that they could never successfully refuse an offer to use substances if faced with this situation. Pay special attention to such members, eliciting group support and suggestions to challenge this pessimistic belief. After the first pair has role-played, ask another pair to go through the same exercise. Depending on the size of the group, continue until everyone has a chance to participate.

With about 8–10 minutes left in the group, you should summarize two or three take-home themes that people should try to remember. You might say something like, "Okay, we're near the end of today's session. Let's summarize the main points we discussed today that people should keep in mind." Encourage people to state two or three major concepts from today's session; when this is done, you should say something like

> "If you only remember a few things from today's group, you should remember the following: that avoiding high-risk situations is the best way to avoid substance use, but sometimes you will be confronted with an offer to use drugs or alcohol. When offered drugs or alcohol, you should use the technique known as 'snapshot versus video thinking' to help you think through your decision. Once you have decided to say 'no,' you should know exactly what you are going to say, and rehearse it so that you can successfully say 'no' when you need to."

You should summarize these main thoughts and write them on the whiteboard, or point them out on the bulletin board and/or Handout 7.1. Make sure that everybody understands these main points, then move onto the skill practice assignment.

Step 5: Distribute Handout 7.2. Review the skill practice for the next group, and ask all members to keep developing and practicing their refusal skills this week (5 minutes).

Congratulate group members for doing a great job in starting to develop these skills, and tell them that it will take much more practice to develop solid refusal skills. Encourage them to refine their answers and to practice them in the upcoming week; tell group members that they will have another chance to role-play in the next group session if they are still struggling with their refusal skills. End the group session by saying that you look forward to seeing them all next week.

Refusing Alcohol and Drugs:
Thinking It Through and Knowing What to Say

Refusing alcohol or drugs is your **last** line of defense against using. Like any last line of defense, you want to use it as little as possible, because if this fails, you are in trouble. Since it **is** your last line of defense, it is most important that your refusal skills be very strong. One major reason that people accept an offer to drink or use drugs, even though they know it is a bad idea, is that they are **unprepared: they don't know what to say**. Therefore, it is important to know exactly what you are going to say, and that you feel comfortable saying it.

   Remember: The single factor that will increase your desire for drugs or alcohol more than anything else is being around alcohol and drugs, including being around people who are using alcohol and drugs. When you are inches away from a drink or a drug, your desire to use it will be stronger than ever. This desire will reduce your ability to think clearly. Even if you hadn't really felt like using beforehand, being offered a drug or a drink may greatly increase your desire. Therefore, you need to **decide** to say no, then know what to say.

   One tool that can help you **decide** to say no is the technique of "snapshot vs. video thinking." People in early recovery often think more about the short-term consequences of their behavior than the long-term consequences. They imagine how a single drink will make them feel, without really thinking about the fact that a "single drink" will turn into two, then four, then eight drinks, and so forth. While **one** drink or **one** line of cocaine may feel good, you know that it won't end there, and that it will end with your feeling much worse, not better. Just thinking about the effect of the **first** drink is what we call "snapshot thinking." **Thinking it through** involves imagining a **video** rather than a **snapshot**. "Watch the whole video" and see how you will feel after four drinks or eight drinks. How will you feel tomorrow? How about the next day? How about the day after that? Imagine how you will feel after you have gone on a binge; most people feel **more** depressed, not less depressed. Imagine how other people might respond to you. Imagine your increased desire to keep drinking if you start with "a drink" tonight. Imagine having to re-set your sobriety date. Continue to say to yourself, "And then what? And then what?" In other words, imagine watching the whole video of all of the consequences of "a drink." That is what **thinking it through** really means: using **video thinking**, not **snapshot thinking**.

   A similar example involves dealing with side effects from medication. If you stop your medication or reduce the dose on your own, you reduce the side effects and may feel better temporarily. But this is just a snapshot—the **short-term** consequence. Now "watch the whole video." Could this increase the likelihood that you'll get more depressed? Could it lead to a manic episode? Romanticizing manic episodes is very common, because **early** mania can feel quite wonderful. That, however, is only the snapshot. "Watch the whole video" and think it through—paranoia, major debts as a result of spending sprees, irritability, and the crashing depression that follows afterward. Just as "having a drink" is a snapshot that will lead to many more drinks and all of the negative consequences that brings, stopping your medication because you like the feeling of early mania will do the same thing. How will you deal with all of the problems that mania will cause? By thinking through the decision and deciding **not** to act as your own doctor, you can avoid disastrous consequences.

   Once you have **decided** to say "no," it is also important to have rehearsed ahead of time **how** you will say "no" to someone who offers you drugs or alcohol; don't count on being able to think of something to say on the spot. Prepare **now**, so that you can get through those high-risk situations when they come up.

   Before reviewing specific things to say, remember that **your best defense against using drugs is to avoid high-risk situations**. What happens, though, when you enter a high-risk situation without realizing it and someone offers you a drink or a drug? What do you say? Here are some general guidelines.

(cont.)

From *Integrated Group Therapy for Bipolar Disorder and Substance Abuse* by Roger D. Weiss and Hilary Smith Connery. Copyright 2011 by The Guilford Press. Permission to photocopy this material is granted to purchasers of this book for personal use only (see copyright page for details).

FIVE RULES TO HELP YOU SAY "NO"

1. **Don't lie**. You don't have to tell the **whole** truth. For example, you don't have to say, "No, thanks, I'm a recovering addict," but you should never lie, because lying will make you nervous and less certain in your response. Also, you may find it hard to remember which lie you said to which people. Remember that recovery involves honesty, both to yourself and to others. You are trying to reestablish your credibility with other people and with yourself. Therefore, don't say anything that is clearly untrue.

2. **You don't have to tell everyone, "I'm a recovering alcoholic/addict."** Your treatment program, including self-help groups (which by now, we hope, you have joined), encourages openness and honesty. For example, at AA meetings, you are encouraged to say, "Hi, my name is 'John,' and I am an alcoholic." Outside of treatment meetings, however, other people may be frightened by alcoholism, drug addiction, and psychiatric illness. Therefore, when dealing with people you don't know or know only casually, or people you know from work, it is not necessary and generally is not a good idea to disclose that the reason you're not drinking is because you are a recovering alcoholic or addict, or that you are taking medication for bipolar disorder. Remember, you can always tell people about these issues later, if you haven't told them so far, but you can never take back what you have already said. **Therefore, if you're not sure whether to reveal something personal about yourself, don't say it now. You can always say it later if you want to do so**.

3. **You can say different things in different situations, as long as what you say is true**. You may want to open up more with friends and family members than with casual acquaintances. You will be seeing them more often, and you don't want to be involved in awkward situations in which they keep asking you about your drinking. It is always safest to avoid being with people who have used alcohol or drugs with you in the past, since trying not to drink or use when they are drinking and using in front of you is **very** difficult—the temptation is just so great. Being with them is an extremely high-risk situation that will act as a trigger to increase your desire to use again.

4. **Don't get upset if someone asks you to drink or use drugs; just refuse calmly**. Don't get angry when someone asks you to drink or use drugs, don't get into an argument, and don't say something that leaves some mystery or bad feeling after you have finished (e.g., don't say, "It's none of your business why I'm not drinking"). You want to be able to say something that ends the conversation firmly but politely, then move on to some other topic.

5. **Say something that you are comfortable saying**. There is no single, standard "best" thing to say when someone asks you whether you want to drink or use drugs. It has to be something that **you feel comfortable** saying. Once you know what you would like to say, practice it until it becomes an automatic response. Below are some examples that have worked for other people.

Sample things to say when asked if you want a drink:

- "I'd love one. Do you have some soda water?"
- "No thanks."
- "No thanks, but do you have something nonalcoholic, like soda water?"
- "No thanks, I'm driving."
- "No thanks, I have to get up early tomorrow."

You may also want to rehearse a strategy for getting out of a social situation in which people are offering you alcohol or drugs:

(cont.)

Sample things to say to escape a high-risk social situation:

- "Excuse me; I forgot to make an important phone call." (This will allow you to step outside in order to leave or to have someone pick you up.)
- "Excuse me; I need to use the rest room." (This will give you time to plan your exit or to place yourself with people who are not using alcohol and drugs.)
- "I forgot to bring my soda; can I get anything for you at the convenience store?" (This allows you either to leave or to return with something safe to drink.)

Sample things to say when asked why you're not drinking alcohol or using drugs:

- "I don't like the way alcohol/using makes me feel lately."
- "I don't like the way I feel the next day after drinking/using."
- "Drinking/using just doesn't agree with me these days."
- "I gave that up."
- "Last time, I had a bad reaction to drinking/using, and I think I'm better off without it."

In general, **you** are going to give much more thought to your alcohol and drug refusal than anyone else will. Most other people don't care one way or another whether you are drinking or using. If someone doesn't ask about your not drinking or using, in general, don't volunteer anything. Just say, "Sure. Can I have some soda water (juice, cola, etc.)?" For many people, refusing an alcoholic drink is easier if they substitute a non-alcoholic drink for it, just so that they are drinking **something**. This is an excellent idea: juice, soda water, soft drinks, and so forth can help you get through a situation like that. Many people find it helpful to arrive at a social gathering prepared with their safe drink of choice; this way the person is in control of pouring himself a nonalcoholic drink. Also, when you are in a restaurant and empty wine glasses have been set at the table (or you are at a wedding and empty champagne glasses are set), you can turn your glass upside down as a signal to the waiter that you do not wish to have any wine poured.

We do *not* recommend substituting nonalcoholic beer or wine. Nonalcoholic beer is not, in fact, completely nonalcoholic. There is a small amount of alcohol in "nonalcoholic" beer. More importantly, though, the process of drinking something that reminds you so much of regular beer (or wine) may serve as a reminder of your past drinking, and may trigger you to want to drink even more. Therefore, nonalcoholic beer or wine is not truly a safe alternative.

SUMMARY

The best way to ensure your recovery is to stay away from high-risk situations; **avoiding situations in which drugs and alcohol are present is *always* your best strategy.** But if you do enter a high-risk situation either by accident or by mistake, that is not the time to figure out what you are going to do or say. You should know ahead of time what you will say if you are offered drugs or alcohol. ***Know* what you are going to say, *practice* it, *rehearse* it,** then hope that you will never have to use it. If you do have to use your refusal skill, this practice exercise could make the difference between staying substance-free and relapsing. Remember, you can maintain recovery as long as you have the **desire** and the **skills** to make it happen.

Skill Practice Homework Sheet: Refusing Alcohol and Drugs: Thinking It Through and Knowing What To Say

Patient Initials: _____

Date: _____

1. What you would say if someone **close** to you (a close friend or a family member) offered you drugs or alcohol?

   _____

   _____

   _____

   _____

2. What you would say if someone that you **didn't** know very well offered you drugs or alcohol?

   _____

   _____

   _____

   _____

3. Write down one plan to escape from an unexpected high-risk situation:

   _____

   _____

   _____

   _____

From *Integrated Group Therapy for Bipolar Disorder and Substance Abuse* by Roger D. Weiss and Hilary Smith Connery. Copyright 2011 by The Guilford Press. Permission to photocopy this material is granted to purchasers of this book for personal use only (see copyright page for details).

SESSION 8

⁐⁐⁐⁐⁐⁐⁐⁐⁐⁐⁐⁐⁐⁐⁐⁐⁐⁐⁐⁐

Using Self-Help Groups

SESSION OBJECTIVES

1. Group members will learn that actively participating in self-help groups increases the likelihood that they will be able to achieve and maintain recovery.

2. Group members will share their own experiences at self-help groups, discussing positive and negative aspects of these experiences.

3. Group members will learn skills to help them to become active members of self-help groups.

MATERIALS REQUIRED

- Bulletin board with the central recovery rule, routes to recovery or relapse, and Session 8 materials posted.
- Dry erase board and markers.
- Copies of Handout 8.1, "Using Self-Help Groups."
- Copies of Handout 8.2, "Skill Practice Homework Sheet: Using Self-Help Groups."

SUMMARY OF SESSION STEPS AND TIME MANAGEMENT

- **Step 1:** Check-in procedure (15 minutes).
- **Step 2:** Review last week's group topic, "Refusing Alcohol and Drugs: Thinking It Through and Knowing What to Say" (5 minutes).

- **Step 3:** Review last week's skill practice questions on Handout 7.2, "Skill Practice Homework Sheet: Refusing Alcohol and Drugs: Thinking It Through and Knowing What to Say" (5 minutes).

- **Step 4:** Distribute Handout 8.1, and discuss the benefits of self-help groups and the challenges to attending them (30 minutes).

    - Benefits and difficulties of alcohol and drug self-help groups.

    - List group members' difficulties, and elicit ways to face these obstacles.

    - Depression and Bipolar Support Alliance support meetings.

- **Step 5:** Distribute Handout 8.2, and ask all members to consider attending a self-help group this week (5 minutes).

BACKGROUND

The primary goal of this group is to have patients discuss their experiences (if any) of attending self-help groups (often called mutual-help or peer-support groups), such as AA, NA, SMART Recovery, Depression and Bipolar Support Alliance (DBSA), and others. The reason a whole group is devoted to this topic is because a good deal of evidence suggests that people who actively use self-help groups are more likely to achieve and maintain recovery than people who don't. Many patients in the group will either be attending self-help groups erratically or not at all, possibly because of negative preconceptions or bad experiences with the groups. The goal of this session is to help patients to identify the benefits of self-help groups; to discuss problems that they have had, or anticipate having, with self-help groups; then to help them solve problems they have identified to facilitate their participation in self-help groups. Group members are taught that participating in self-help groups improves their chances of successful recovery.

Step 1: Check-in procedure (15 minutes).

Following the group leaders' announcements (e.g., expected member or leader absences, changes to the group meeting schedule or site, introductions for new members), all patients should review their weekly progress according to Handout 1.2, "Monitoring Your Symptoms: How to Check In on Your Recovery" (see Session 1). During this time, other group members are discouraged from commenting on the individual's check-in report, since relevant discussions can occur during the review of the skill practice. The group leaders should make brief summary comments that recognize and positively reinforce any thought or behavioral changes that indicate that the group members are making efforts to achieve abstinence and mood stability or to directly apply the central recovery rule. Check-in is also a time for the group leaders to listen carefully for any content that might provide a useful opportunity for the group to discuss this week's group theme; for this session, leaders will note any reports of group members' participation in self-help groups in the past week, and ask about those experiences.

Step 2: Review last week's group topic, "Refusing Alcohol and Drugs: Thinking It Through and Knowing What to Say" (5 minutes).

Ask group members how they did this week with developing drink- and drug-refusal skills and how much they practiced these. Ask if any members had a hard time with this, and have other group members provide helpful feedback to those individuals. Ask if any group members actually had to use their refusal skills last week, and inquire how that turned out. Ask if anyone used the "snapshot versus video thinking" technique, and ask how that worked out. If someone was unsuccessful in using the "snapshot versus video" technique or the refusal skills, and used drugs or alcohol, ask the group members to give that person feedback about how he or she might have better success next time.

Step 3: Review last week's skill practice questions on Handout 7.2, "Skill Practice Homework Sheet: Refusing Alcohol and Drugs: Thinking It Through and Knowing What to Say" (5 minutes).

Make note of instances in which group members' refusal responses were different with people close to them versus with acquaintances. Make sure that everyone has had a chance to develop a good "escape plan" when faced with a high-risk situation.

Step 4: Distribute Handout 8.1, and discuss the benefits of self-help groups and the challenges to attending them (30 minutes).

Announce today's topic: "Using Self-Help Groups." Say that one thing we know about alcohol and drug abuse self-help groups is that people who actively participate in them generally have a greater chance of recovery than do those who don't use them. Tell them that this is why an entire session is devoted to this topic—to help members to think about what might prevent them from actively participating in a self-help group, and about what they might do differently that would make it easier to participate in a self-help group.

Benefits and difficulties of alcohol and drug self-help groups.

Then say, "How many people here have been to alcohol or drug self-help groups?" After people raise their hands, you can then ask, "Who has been to self-help groups in the past *week*?" Most likely, fewer people will raise their hands. Pay attention to the people who raise their hands after the first question but not after the second question. Among people who have been to self-help groups in the past week, ask which ones they have been to and write them down on the board. Whenever someone mentions a particular group (e.g., AA), ask which *other* people have been to AA. Go through all of the groups that people have attended in the past week, then ask whether people have attended *other* self-help groups in the past, until all of the major self-help groups have been mentioned. Then come back to the people who have been to self-help groups in the past, but not in the last week, and ask whether there was a reason they didn't go in the last week. Most likely, they will either say that they didn't like them or give some personal reason (e.g., "I didn't have the energy to go"). You might then say something like "So not everybody goes to self-help groups; there are obviously some problems. We are here to discuss and figure out how to overcome these problems. First, let's talk about what people see as the benefits of self-help groups." Then make a list on the board. These items could include the following: role modeling, optimism, education about the illness, practical advice about staying clean and sober, development of drug-free relationships, support, availability of the groups, the fact that they are free, the availability of the wisdom of other people, the fact that some people find the program philosophy comforting, the structure that such groups provide, social contact, a concrete guide to recovery, and recognition for the hard work that is part of recovery. People may come up with other benefits as well.

List group members' difficulties, and elicit ways to face these obstacles.

Then ask people what kinds of *problems* they have had going to self-help meetings. These may be divided into several types of problems:

1. Problems with the *philosophy* of 12-step meetings (an objection to the idea of a Higher Power, an objection to the spiritual nature of the program, a sense that the program is simplistic and rigid, an objection to the notions of powerlessness and surrender).
2. Some people may object to the *people* they meet in addiction self-help meetings: they don't relate to the people, perhaps because other people don't have BD or they are of different age, gender, social class, and so forth.
3. People may have difficulties with meetings for reasons not intrinsic to the meetings themselves, but because they have difficulty mobilizing themselves to get to meetings, perhaps because of depression or more practical problems, such as difficulty with transportation or child care. Fear of stigma is also a stumbling block for many patients—the fear of who will see them at the meeting.

Next, say, "Let's talk about how to deal with some of the problems that people have brought up." You can then divide these into (1) problems with the *program* (i.e., the 12 steps, spirituality, the Higher Power), (2) problems with the *people* (not feeling that you can relate to other people in the program), and (3) problems with yourself (you have no objection to going, but you are having difficulty mobilizing yourself or are having some of the practical problems mentioned earlier). Then you can say, "Let's start with problems with the *program*: people who object to the idea of spirituality or a Higher Power (or whatever else people have brought up). Are there people in the group who have managed to solve these problems or overcome them?" Then you can take suggestions from other group members about how to deal with these problems. Potential ways to think about this include the following:

1. People don't need to "buy into" the entire program to get a great deal out of self-help meetings. Many people who are turned off by the concept of a Higher Power go to AA or NA meetings for the fellowship, practical advice, structure, socialization, and so forth. Emphasize that, as a large group program, not everything in the program will be directly relevant to every person that goes. One thing you might say is,

"If you spend an hour and a half at an AA meeting, you may find that you get one really positive thing from it, that there are many things that you disagree with, and that a large number of things said are things you don't really agree or disagree with but are sort of irrelevant to you. But if you learned one important thing from the meeting, it's probably time better spent than almost anything else you would have done during that hour and a half."

2. You should let people know that SMART Recovery is a non-12-step alternative self-help group that does not include the concept of a Higher Power and is not spiritual. SMART Recovery also does not use sponsors. The meetings tend to be relatively small. While this group has some appeal, one potential disadvantage is the fact that it tends to have fewer people with long-term sobriety. However, people who don't like 12-step meetings should certainly try SMART Recovery, Women for Sobriety, or Save Our Selves (SOS)—all examples of non-12-step self-help groups.

3. Some people with BD object to 12-step meetings, because they have heard from certain people in AA or NA that they shouldn't be taking medication. While this happens much less now than in the past, this is an important issue to address directly. Emphasize that official AA publications, including one entitled "The AA Member—Medications and Other Drugs," are very clear about advocating that people follow their doctor's advice regarding medication. AA *in no way* recommends stopping medication. Some people in AA may make such recommendations, but that is only because AA is composed of lots of different people: some who have terrific ideas, and others whose ideas are quite unhelpful. If a person goes to an AA meeting and finds that the vast majority of attendees are unsympathetic toward people having to take medication, he or she should go to a different meeting.

Another objection some people have to 12-step meetings is they hear that they need to go to "90 meetings in 90 days," or be criticized by other members for not going to enough meetings. It is important to emphasize that *consistency* of attendance is more important than the actual *number* of meetings someone attends. It is preferable to follow through on one's commitment to go than to make unrealistic and lofty goals, then not follow through on them. In other words, it is better to pledge to go to one meeting a week and do it than to pledge to go to six meetings a week and go to only three.

5. *Participation* in meetings is also useful. Participation does not necessarily mean talking in meetings. It can also mean reading AA or SMART Recovery literature, talking to someone from AA outside of a meeting, having a 12-step sponsor (particularly helpful), making coffee at a meeting, and so forth. Research has shown that people who participate at meetings do better than those who just go and don't participate in any way.

6. People who have difficulty with the *fellowship* (i.e., they don't relate to the people that they have met in 12-step meetings) should be encouraged to "shop around" for meetings: *finding the right match*.

7. You can help people who have difficulty with some of the *practical* aspects of self-help meetings to problem-solve around issues of transportation, child care, and so forth: finding meetings accessible by public transportation, meetings in which child care is provided, or going to a meeting at a different time of day when child care is less of an issue, and so forth. As the group ends, tell people that you would like everyone to go to at least one self-help group this week, and to try to use some of the principles the group talked about today in overcoming some of their problems related to self-help groups.

Depression and Bipolar Support Alliance meetings.

Then say, "We started out talking about alcohol and drug self-help groups like AA and NA. How many people have gone to DBSA—Depression and Bipolar Support Alliance (formerly called Manic-Depressive and Depressive Association, or MDDA)? How about groups like Double Trouble or Dual Recovery Anonymous, which are designed for people with both substance abuse problems and psychiatric illness?" Depending on the availability of these meetings in your area, you may have many members attending them regularly or no members who are even familiar with these groups. If DBSA is available in your region, encourage group members to try attending it, since many people who attend DBSA meetings have both BD (or at least experience with depression) and substance abuse problems. Even if it is not in your area, members can go to the DBSA website (*www.dbsalliance.org*) for useful information and online supports. Similarly, Double Trouble and Dual Recovery Anonymous may be very helpful, depending on the availability and strength of these groups in your geographic area.

With about 8–10 minutes left in the session, you should summarize two or three take-home themes that people should try to remember. You might say something like "Okay, we're near the end of today's group. Let's summarize the main points we discussed today that people should keep in mind." Encourage people to state two or three major concepts from today's session; when this is done, you should say something like "If you only remember two things from today's group, you should remember the following: that self-help groups can be very helpful to you in your recovery, and that even though you may have some problems with these groups, you can deal with those problems." You should summarize these main thoughts and write them on the whiteboard, or point them out on the bulletin board and/or the session topic Handout 8.1. Make sure that everybody understands these main points, then move on to the skill practice assignment.

Step 5: Distribute Handout 8.2, and ask all members to consider attending a self-help group this week (5 minutes).

Ask group members to think about what they like and don't like about self-help groups, and how they can overcome challenges dealing with self-help groups. Remind them that attending self-help groups improves their chances of a successful recovery. End the group by saying that you look forward to seeing them all next week.

Using Self-Help Groups

BENEFITS OF SELF-HELP GROUPS

- There is a lot of wisdom at self-help meetings. Many people at these groups who have been in the same or similar position to the one you are in are now doing well. It is useful to find out how they did it.

- Meetings can give you hope. You will see people who were in such terrible shape that it seems like a miracle that they now are doing so well. If they can do it, so can you.

- You will probably learn more in an Alcoholics Anonymous (AA), Narcotics Anonymous (NA), or Depression and Bipolar Support Alliance (DBSA) meeting than you would if you did something else during that hour and a half. It is important to realize that, like any large group, some of the things you hear at a meeting will be irrelevant to you; some advice will be frankly harmful, some will be only slightly relevant, and some will be just right. Listen for the things that are just right and learn from them. If there are things said that are irrelevant or wrong for you, reject or politely ignore them.

- You will find other people there who are like you—if not right away, then later on. If you don't find them at the meeting you have been attending, try going to another meeting. Different meetings may be very different from each other, so don't give up on meetings just because you don't like one particular meeting you attended.

- AA, NA, and DBSA remind you of some very basic issues: (1) Your life will be better off if you don't drink or use drugs; (2) your life will be worse if you start using drugs or alcohol again, or if you keep using; (3) you can stop using drugs and alcohol; (4) you can stay clean and sober; (5) staying clean and sober can improve your mood; and (6) you are not responsible for your illnesses but you are responsible for your recovery. DBSA also offers very practical support and information about bipolar disorder that may help you in management of the illness.

- Self-help groups offer fellowship: people in self-help groups support each other in a different way than do friends, family, or professionals. They have a different understanding from anyone else about what you're going through. Asking people at meetings to help you helps them as well, which is why they help you. When you are feeling alone and desperate, and feel as if you're about to drink or get high, you can call someone. What's more, that person will *want* you to call, and won't get mad or say "There you go again"; this understanding and acceptance can make the difference between your using versus staying clean and sober. When you're tempted to stop your medication, someone from DBSA will be happy to remind you of the consequences.

THINGS YOU MAY NOT LIKE ABOUT SELF-HELP GROUPS

- You may feel as if you are walking into a "club" in which everyone else knows each other, yet you don't know anyone, anything, or even the rules.

- You may see lots of people hugging each other, yet no one is saying hello to you.

- On the other hand, you may find people that you barely know coming up to hug you, which may make you feel uncomfortable. You may hear talk about God, spirituality, and a Higher Power that may turn you off. You may hear people talking about giving up substances and having their lives turn around, while you may have given up substances and find yourself still struggling with symptoms of bipolar disorder.

(cont.)

From *Integrated Group Therapy for Bipolar Disorder and Substance Abuse* by Roger D. Weiss and Hilary Smith Connery. Copyright 2011 by The Guilford Press. Permission to photocopy this material is granted to purchasers of this book for personal use only (see copyright page for details).

- You may hear phrases at AA that seem insensitive, such as "Take the cotton out of your ears and stick it in your mouth." You may be offended by the language.
- Some people in addiction self-help groups may criticize the idea of psychiatry, therapy, or taking medication.
- You may be told that you are "sitting on the pity pot" if you talk about being depressed at an AA or NA meeting.
- You may be told at an AA or NA meeting that if you are still feeling depressed despite being clean and sober, you are not doing your program right—that you're not going to enough meetings or speaking up enough.
- You may be told that you need to go to 90 meetings in 90 days, when it is not possible for you to do so.
- You may feel embarrassed going to an AA, NA, or DBSA meeting, and worry about who will see you there.
- You may find that some SMART Recovery groups focus more on criticizing AA than on promoting recovery.
- You may worry about people waiting outside groups, or even attending groups, who are really there to try to get other people to drink or use drugs with them.

OVERCOMING THESE PROBLEMS

Why go to self-help groups when they have all of these potential problems? Reread all of the reasons listed under "Benefits of Self-Help Groups." Remember, you will probably learn more in a self-help meeting than you would doing almost anything else during that hour and a half. If you hear things in a meeting that you don't like, politely ignore them. Not everything you hear in these meetings will be absolutely appropriate to you, but if you listen actively during a meeting, you will most likely hear something that is very valuable to you.

Be choosy about the people you spend time with at meetings: as you would anywhere else, look for others who are committed to sobriety and improving their lives. If someone is making you feel uncomfortable, get a little distance from him or her or make an effort to meet other people at the meeting.

If you find that you simply don't like the 12-step program, consider SMART Recovery, a non-12-step self-help group. If you feel that you can't relate to the people you meet in a particular AA or DBSA meeting, try another AA or DBSA meeting. Try lots of different meetings. Remember that going to a self-help meeting is like going to a restaurant. You know that you will be served food there, but each restaurant is otherwise different. Each AA meeting is different. Each DBSA meeting is also different. Shop around. If available, try large meetings, small meetings, all-male or all-female meetings, open meetings, closed meetings, and step meetings. At the beginning, it is often helpful to attend Beginners' AA or NA meetings until you feel comfortable enough to attend other meetings. See what you like and don't like. Read the literature that is available or given to you. Then make a commitment to go to a certain number of meetings you like each week. The number is not nearly as important as the fact that you have made a commitment and are following through on it. It is better to commit to two meetings a week and **go to both of them** than to commit to seven meetings a week and go to only five.

Staying clean and sober is about making a commitment and following through on it, not about making grand promises and following through only part way. Self-help groups can help in that way. Remember that the goal is to stay clean and sober, and learn to manage your bipolar disorder, so that your life will get better; self-help groups can help to accomplish those aims.

Skill Practice Homework Sheet: Using Self-Help Groups

Patient Initials: _____

Date: _____

1. Name two things that you like about self-help groups.

   _____

   _____

2. Name two things that you do not like about self-help groups.

   _____

   _____

   For the items that you do not like, what could you do to overcome those problems?

   _____

   _____

3. What would you do if someone told you at an AA or NA meeting that you should stop taking your medication?

   _____

   _____

4. What would you do if someone at an NA meeting told you that he or she was still using and could get you some drugs?

   _____

   _____

5. What would you say to someone you didn't know well who kept asking you for things, such as your phone number or rides to meetings?

   _____

   _____

   _____

From *Integrated Group Therapy for Bipolar Disorder and Substance Abuse* by Roger D. Weiss and Hilary Smith Connery. Copyright 2011 by The Guilford Press. Permission to photocopy this material is granted to purchasers of this book for personal use only (see copyright page for details).

SESSION 9

Taking Medication

SESSION OBJECTIVES

1. Group members will share their personal experiences of both the benefits and the problems with taking medications.

2. Group members will share their difficulties with medication adherence and understand that medications for BD and for SUD only work well if they are faithfully taken as prescribed every day.

3. Group members will learn how to keep a *medication log*, which achieves three goals:

   a. Improve medication adherence.

   b. Monitor side effects.

   c. Monitor changes in target symptoms.

4. Group members will learn that bringing their medication log to appointments with their prescribing doctor or nurse is a highly effective way to develop a collaborative relationship with their prescriber and to achieve the best results from medication trials or adjustments.

MATERIALS REQUIRED

- Bulletin board with the central recovery rule, routes to recovery or relapse, and Session 9 materials posted.

- Dry erase board and markers.

- Copies of Handout 9.1, "Taking Medication," including the sample medication log.

- Copies of Handout 9.2, "Skill Practice Homework Sheet: Taking Medication."

SUMMARY OF SESSION STEPS AND TIME MANAGEMENT

- **Step 1:** Check-in procedure (15 minutes).
- **Step 2:** Review last week's group topic, "Using Self-Help Groups" (5 minutes).
- **Step 3:** Review last week's skill practice questions on Handout 8.2, "Skill Practice Homework Sheet: Using Self-Help Groups" (5 minutes).
- **Step 4:** Distribute Handout 9.1, and discuss the benefits and challenges of taking medications and monitoring medication intake (30 minutes).
  - Discuss the challenges of taking medications for bipolar disorder.
  - Demonstrate that thoughts about medication can lead to nonadherent behavior.
  - Group members assess their beliefs about and the practice of taking medication.
  - Discuss how skills from "Denial, Ambivalence, and Acceptance" (Session 5) apply to taking medication.
  - Group members create a "pros and cons" square for taking medication.
  - Common benefits and problems with taking medication.
  - Taking too much medication.
  - Communication with prescribing clinicians is essential and is aided by a medication log.
  - How to fill out the medication log.
- **Step 6:** Distribute Handout 9.2, and ask all members to make a medication log and keep a daily calendar of their medication adherence, benefits, or problems (5 minutes).

BACKGROUND

This session encourages group members to resolve ambivalent thoughts they may have about having to take medication for BD. The group reviews the many benefits of taking medication, as well as common problems with taking medications. In fact, adherence to prescribed medication is so essential to recovery that it is included as part of the central recovery rule; virtually all patients diagnosed with BD require ongoing medication for recovery. Members are encouraged and empowered to develop an active role by collaborating with their prescribing doctor or nurse; keeping a log of medication side effects, as well as changes in target symptoms; and bringing this with them to appointments. Group members are taught that patients with BD frequently require several different medication trials before arriving at the combination of medications that result in the "best fit" for maintenance—both tolerable and effective at controlling BD symptoms. It is common for patients with BD to feel frustrated about having to try medication after medication, so it is important for group leaders to normalize this (pharmacological genetics may provide future improvements to this process). It is emphasized that taking medication is an essential part of recovery, and that, on the whole, the benefits of taking medication outweigh the burdens.

A word of advice: Don't allow group members to talk too much about their specific medication questions. Rather, encourage them to bring individual concerns to their prescribing nurse or doctor. At times, patients may bring up negative feelings toward their nurse or doctor, such as doubts about their competence or complaints about their unavailability, style, or manner. This can be tricky, but in the group setting, it is best to advise members to bring up such concerns with their prescribing clinician, saying that, in the majority of cases, talking about such concerns directly can lead to improvement in the situation. Advising patients about the possibility and benefits of consultation for a second opinion may sometimes be helpful or appropriate in this situation. It is important to tell members explicitly that they should never stop taking medication based only on their belief that their prescribing clinician is making a wrong decision, or is perceived to be unavailable; emphasize that it is very dangerous behavior to "be your own doctor" with BD medications.

Step 1: Check-in procedure (15 minutes).

Following the group leaders' announcements (e.g., expected member or leader absences, changes to the group meeting schedule or site, introductions for new members), all patients should review their weekly progress according to Handout 1.2, "Monitoring Your Symptoms: How to Check In on Your Recovery" (see Session 1). During this time, other group members are discouraged from commenting on the individual's check-in report, since relevant discussions can occur during the review of the skill practice. The group leaders should make brief summary comments that recognize and positively reinforce any thought or behavioral changes that indicate that the group members are making efforts to achieve abstinence and mood stability or to directly apply the central recovery rule. Check-in is also a time for the group leaders to listen carefully for any content that might provide a useful opportunity for the group to discuss this week's group theme; for this session, leaders note any reports of missed medication doses or problems with medication adherence.

Step 2: Review last week's group topic, "Using Self-Help Groups" (5 minutes).

Ask group members whether they attended a new self-help group during the past week or participated more actively in a group they were already attending. Ask members whether the discussion in last week's group helped to make them more comfortable or open-minded about using self-help groups. If not, try to find out what is causing members to continue to struggle, and help them to think of solutions. Remind group members that using self-help groups greatly increases their chances of achieving and maintaining recovery, and also provides social relationships with other people facing similar issues.

Step 3: Review last week's skill practice questions on Handout 8.2, "Skill Practice Homework Sheet: Using Self-Help Groups" (5 minutes).

Pay careful attention to the answers that involve members setting interpersonal limits, since these skills are often difficult for people with BD. If a member reports difficulty with social interactions at self-help groups, consider doing some brief role plays that help to model appropriate communication skills and behaviors.

Step 4: Distribute Handout 9.1, and discuss the benefits and challenges of taking medications and monitoring medication intake (30 minutes).

Discuss the challenges of taking medications for bipolar disorder.

Announce today's topic: "Taking Medication." Tell the group,

> "We are spending a whole session talking about taking medication, because it can be very difficult to take medication as prescribed. Medications come with a variety of problems, yet they are necessary for recovery from bipolar disorder. So the goal today is to figure out the best ways to lessen the burdens of bipolar disorder medications, so that taking medication is more comfortable and effective. People with bipolar disorder have different reasons for not taking their medication as prescribed. Can you name any?"

Write group members' examples on the board. If the following reasons are not stated, add these: "Sometimes when you're feeling good or a little too good (i.e., hypomanic), you don't want to take any medication, because you feel you don't need it. Other times, when you feel depressed, you may want to take too much medication, because you feel desperate to change the way you feel. Or maybe you want to stop taking medication altogether, because you just feel like giving up."

Demonstrate that thoughts about medication can lead to nonadherent behavior.

From the responses on the board, circle the ones that are *thoughts* about medications, and demonstrate how these thoughts lead to the behavior of skipping doses or stopping medication. *Common thoughts leading to poor medication adherence* include (1) ambivalence about whether one believes that one has BD, (2) a negative attitude or belief about medication maintenance (e.g., "I only need to take medication when I am depressed" or "When it comes down to it, I just don't like taking pills"), (3) thoughts or fears about medication side effects (e.g., "I know that divalproex makes people fat," "I don't want medication to change my personality"), or (4) a belief that "if a little is good, then more is better," which can lead people to take *more* medication than prescribed.

Group members assess their beliefs about and the practice of taking medication.

Next, ask members to go around the room and verbally report their answers to the following two questions:

1. "On a scale of 0–100, how much do you believe that you need to take medication for BD? A score of 100 means that you absolutely believe you need medication, while a score of 0 means that you are absolutely sure that you don't need medication."
2. "What percentage of time in the previous 6 months have you taken your medication as prescribed?"

The majority of people will respond very positively to the first question, and somewhat less so on the second. Rarely, someone will give a higher score on the second question. Both patterns are worth noting.

Discuss how skills from "Denial, Ambivalence, and Acceptance" (Session 5) apply to taking medication.

When there is a disparity between these two answers, particularly in the direction of a higher score on the first question, review some of the skills from the session Handout 5.1, "Denial, Ambivalence, and Acceptance," and apply these to taking medication every day. Tell group members,

> "It is important to work on acceptance of the need for taking medication for bipolar disorder, because if you don't accept this, and you just react passively by forgetting your medication or letting it run out without refilling it, you will resolve your ambivalence by 'hitting bottom' and having a disastrous experience. That's a terrible way to learn about the importance of taking your medication as prescribed."

If a group member has done this in the past, invite that individual to share with the group the consequences and costs of learning the hard way, to reinforce the point.

Group members create a "pros and cons" square for taking medication.

Now say, "One safe way for people to resolve their ambivalence about taking medication is to complete a 'pros and cons square,' which you will do now in group and also as part of your skill practice homework this week." Draw the following pros and cons square on the board:

Subject of ambivalence:	PRO	CON
Taking medication as prescribed		
NOT taking medication as prescribed		

Select a volunteer from the group to fill in the pros and cons square for his or her medication situation. If another person volunteers, repeat this process for that group member as well. Teach them that weighing the pros and cons of a topic they feel unsure about is a great way to think about a problem, because they get a lot of clear information on paper to consider and can identify how well the pros outweigh the cons. When they do, you can resolve in favor of the pros, deciding that it is worth it to take medication. If the cons outweigh the pros, group members may need to consider an alternative path, in this case, speaking with their prescribing clinician about a medication change. Tell them that no matter what they decide on their own, *never change or stop medications before discussing the issue with their prescriber!*

Common benefits and problems with taking medication.

The group may also review common benefits and problems associated with taking medication, as listed in Handout 9.1. The *benefits of taking medication* are:

- Avoid psychosis.
- Avoid hospitalization.
- Reduce your likelihood of substance use.
- Make yourself feel more responsible by taking care of yourself.
- Avoid manic spending sprees.
- Avoid depression.
- Improve your sleep.
- Avoid risky sexual behaviors.
- Make yourself feel that you're doing all that you can do for yourself.
- Make other people in your life feel that you're doing all that you can do for yourself.
- Avoid the potential negative impact on your friends/family if you become manic, psychotic, or very depressed.
- Make yourself less irritable and more patient with yourself and other people.
- Avoid losing a job or failing in school.
- Avoid legal problems.
- Avoid accidents (car crashes due to reckless driving or driving under the influence) and injuries.
- Personal or individual benefits specific to your situation.

Unfortunately, *medications also present problems to people*, which can be divided into three major types:

- Side effects
- Effects on mood or thought
- Difficulties accepting a lifelong illness and the need to take medication for it

Common medication side effects include weight gain, headache, cognitive impairment (slowed thinking, confusion, poor memory), tremor, nausea, diarrhea, dry mouth, blurred vision, reduced sexual drive, hair loss, sleepiness, "jitteriness," feeling "spaced out," increased sweating, and the need to have blood drawn. It is important to note that side effects are different for different people, and a particular side effect that may represent a mere annoyance to one person may be profoundly disturbing to someone else.

Taking too much medication.

Not all forms of medication nonadherence involve taking too *little* medication. Some people with BD and SUD take *more* medication than prescribed. Some such situations are unsurprising (e.g., taking benzodiazepines such as lorazepam [Ativan], clonazepam [Klonopin], or alprazolam [Xanax] in higher doses than prescribed. However, we have also found in our research that patients with BD and SUD frequently take medications without abuse potential in greater doses than prescribed. The most common reason for this is impatience, waiting for the medication to work. Therefore, someone who is prescribed 20 mg a day of fluoxetine (Prozac) might take 40 or 60 mg on a day that he or she is particularly depressed. This type of "self-medication" can lead to problems similar to those encountered when people decide to stop their medication or take a reduced dose. Thus, it is useful to ask here, "Who has taken *more* medication than prescribed?" If people report having done this, ask what led them to do it. Then say that better communication with the prescribing doctor or nurse can help one reduce the temptation to be one's own doctor.

Communication with prescribing clinicians is essential and is aided by a medication log.

The use of medication should be a collaborative effort between a patient and his or her doctor or nurse. *Many people with BD require several medication changes or combinations before they get a "good fit" that works well for them and that they can tolerate taking daily.* Tell the group, "The only way to find the right medication(s) for you is to ask your doctor how the medication you are going to take works, what symptoms are expected to improve with the medication, what side effects are common, and whether there are any potential dangers you need to know about your medication (e.g., lithium toxicity)." Since this is a lot of information to handle, encourage group members to ask their doctor or nurse to write down three things for them: (1) what symptoms should get better with this medication, (2) common side effects, and (3) safety issues that would be a reason to call the doctor or nurse immediately. With this information at hand, group members can begin taking the medication while keeping a medication log that keeps track of whether they remembered to take their medication, whether their symptoms improved, and any new side effects they noticed (a blank medication log is distributed with Handout 9.1).

How to fill out the medication log.

Group members should bring this log to every appointment with their prescribing clinician. Illustrated below is a sample medication log that has been filled out:

Medication	Date started	Missed doses?	Target symptoms	Side effects
Divalproex 1500 mg night	01/01/2010	no	Racing thoughts are better	Weight gain 5 lbs.
Risperidone 2 mg a.m./p.m.	02/01/2010	3 days forgot my morning dose	Paranoid thoughts have gone away	A little sleepy during the day but it's OK
Trazodone 100 mg night	01/01/2010	no	Still having trouble getting to sleep	None

Use the dry erase board and this sample log to show group members how to keep a summary log of medications being taken, how well they are working, and side effects. Suggest that the use of a pill box can help them to be organized about their medications.

With about 8–10 minutes left in the group, you should summarize two or three take-home themes that people should try to remember. You might say something like "Okay, we're near the end of today's group. Let's summarize the main points we discussed today that people should keep in mind." Encourage people to state two or three major concepts from today's session; when this is done, you should say something like "If you only remember a few things from today's group, you should remember the following: that medication has both benefits and problems, but the benefits ordinarily outweigh the problems. If you are having problems, talk to your prescriber about them, don't try to be your own doctor." You should summarize these main thoughts and write them on the whiteboard, or point them out on the bulletin board and/or the session topic Handout 9.1. Make sure that everybody understands these main points, then move on to the skill practice assignment.

Step 5: Distribute Handout 9.2, and ask all members to make a medication log and keep a daily calendar of their medication adherence, benefits, or problems (5 minutes).

Review the skill practice for the next session. Tell group members that you look forward to seeing them next week, when there will be time to review their success using these recovery skills.

Taking Medication

Many people with bipolar disorder consider the idea of not taking their medication as prescribed at some time during their lives. Accepting the need for ongoing medication treatment comes more easily for some people than for others; some struggle for months or years with the idea of taking medication. Unfortunately, not taking medication properly generally leads to disastrous consequences: a return of bipolar disorder symptoms, relapse to substance abuse, hospitalization, and overall life disruption.

In general, people take their medication as prescribed for a straightforward reason: They believe that the benefits of taking medication are greater than the problems involved with not taking it. People who don't take their medication, on the other hand, believe the opposite: that the problems outweigh the good. This handout is designed to help you become and remain more aware of the benefits of taking prescribed medication and to minimize some of the problems that can be caused by taking medications.

BENEFITS OF TAKING MEDICATION

- Avoid psychosis.
- Avoid hospitalization.
- Reduce your likelihood of substance use.
- Make yourself feel more responsible by taking care of yourself.
- Avoid manic spending sprees.
- Avoid depression.
- Improve your sleep.
- Avoid risky sexual behaviors.
- Make yourself feel that you're doing all that you can do for yourself.
- Make other people in your life feel that you're doing all that you can do for yourself.
- Avoid the potential negative impact on your friends/family if you become manic, psychotic, or very depressed.
- Make yourself less irritable and more patient with yourself and other people.
- Avoid losing a job or failing in school.
- Avoid legal problems.
- Avoid accidents (car crashes due to reckless driving or driving under the influence) and injuries.
- Personal or individual benefits specific to your situation.

(cont.)

From *Integrated Group Therapy for Bipolar Disorder and Substance Abuse* by Roger D. Weiss and Hilary Smith Connery. Copyright 2011 by The Guilford Press. Permission to photocopy this material is granted to purchasers of this book for personal use only (see copyright page for details).

PROBLEMS WITH TAKING MEDICATION

Unfortunately, medications also present problems to people, which can be divided into three major types:

- Side effects
- Effects on mood or thought
- Difficulties accepting that you have a lifelong illness and need to take medication for it

SUGGESTIONS FOR DEALING WITH THESE PROBLEMS

Side Effects

Like all medications, mood stabilizers, antidepressants, and antipsychotic drugs have their share of side effects; these are different for different people and vary in how much they bother people. Some side effects can be dealt with by changing the dose; by adding another medication; by certain physical treatments (e.g., support stockings for leg swelling); by taking the medications at different times of the day; or, in some instances, by stopping a medication and/or switching to a different medication. Some people don't like to "bother" their doctor with their lists of side effects, so they suffer silently. This often continues until they can't stand it any more, then simply stop taking the medication. Obviously, this does them no good. We strongly recommend that you keep a medication log (see below) as the best way of working with your prescribing doctor or nurse to find the right medication or combinations of medications for your recovery. You may need to try several medications before finding the one that works best for you. Have patience! Your recovery is worth it.

Watch out for the opposite problem, too—taking **more** medication than prescribed. The two most common reasons people do this are (1) impatience with waiting for the medication to work and (2) the belief that "more is better." Talking with your prescriber about the **amount** of medication you should take can help you to avoid the problems of "being your own doctor."

During your appointment, ask your prescribing doctor or nurse to help you understand any new medication you will be starting by writing down (1) what symptoms should get better with this medication, (2) common side effects, and (3) safety issues that would be a reason to call your prescriber right away. This way, you have a record of this information, so you don't have to worry about forgetting what you have been told that day. Now, it's up to you to keep a **medication log** that keeps track of how well the medication is working for you. We have included a blank medication log at the end of this handout.

You may want to use a pillbox to organize your medications for the week, so that you don't miss doses. When you go to your follow-up appointments with your doctor or nurse, bring your medication log with you, so that together you can review whether you have been taking your medication regularly enough to be effective, whether your target symptoms are improving, and any new side effects you have noticed.

Effects on Mood or Thought

Sometimes people worry that taking medication dulls their creativity, makes them less fun to be around, changes their personality in a negative way, or makes them "less sharp" in their thinking. If you believe that your medication is affecting you in any of these ways, write down what you are worried about, then talk it over with your doctor or nurse. You might also talk it over with family and friends to see whether what you are experiencing is noticeable to anyone else.

(cont.)

138

Lack of Acceptance

As we discussed in the Session on "Denial, Ambivalence, and Acceptance," acceptance involves coming to terms with your bipolar disorder and your substance use disorder, understanding that you need to do whatever you can to treat them both properly, and believing that your life is okay anyway. Achieving acceptance is difficult and generally involves connecting with people. This can be done in therapy, in this group, with friends and family, and through self-help groups such as AA, NA, SMART Recovery, Dual Recovery Anonymous, Double Trouble, and Depression and Bipolar Support Alliance (DBSA). Talking with other people who have seen you when your mood symptoms were uncontrolled can help if you notice you are having denial thoughts ("Maybe I'm better now; maybe I don't need this medication anymore"). Remember that denial is characterized by "blind spots," so you definitely need someone else to see things in yourself that you can't see because of these blind spots.

   Although you know that taking medication is necessary, you may someday find yourself trying to talk yourself out of doing what you know in your heart you should do. If this happens, it is likely that one of the problems described earlier is involved. By using some of the actions mentioned in this handout, you will be able to talk yourself back into doing the right thing, and taking care of yourself.

(cont.)

Medication Log

Medication	Date started	Missed doses?	Target symptoms	Side effects

From *Integrated Group Therapy for Bipolar Disorder and Substance Abuse* by Roger D. Weiss and Hilary Smith Connery. Copyright 2011 by The Guilford Press. Permission to photocopy this material is granted to purchasers of this book for personal use only (see copyright page for details).

Skill Practice Homework Sheet: Taking Medication

Patient Initials: _____

Date: _____

1. Please list below two benefits of taking medications for bipolar disorder.

   _____

   _____

2. Name two feelings, thoughts, side effects, or situations that have gotten in the way of taking your medications.

   _____

   _____

3. What positive action will you take this week to help you take your medications? Be specific, so that you can tell clearly whether you are following through on your plan.

   _____

   _____

4. Complete the following pros and cons square for taking your medications. What does it tell you?

	PRO	CON
Taking medication as prescribed		
NOT taking medication as prescribed		

From *Integrated Group Therapy for Bipolar Disorder and Substance Abuse* by Roger D. Weiss and Hilary Smith Connery. Copyright 2011 by The Guilford Press. Permission to photocopy this material is granted to purchasers of this book for personal use only (see copyright page for details).

◯◯◯◯◯◯◯◯◯◯◯◯◯◯◯◯◯◯

Recovery versus Relapse Thinking

It Matters What You Do

SESSION OBJECTIVES

1. Group members are reminded that thoughts lead to behaviors; recovery thoughts lead to recovery behaviors, while relapse thoughts lead to relapse behaviors.

2. Group members will learn to identify "may as well" thinking, discuss examples of "may as well" thinking, and understand that "may as well" thinking is often an example of either substance use thinking or depressive (or sometimes manic) thinking.

3. Group members will learn the technique called "hang up on your disease" as a way of countering "may as well" thinking.

4. Group members will learn that what they choose to do *always* matters to their recovery.

MATERIALS REQUIRED

- Bulletin board with the central recovery rule, routes to recovery or relapse, and Session 10 materials posted.
- Dry erase board and markers.
- Copies of Handout 10.1, "Recovery versus Relapse Thinking."
- Copies of Handout 10.2, "Skill Practice Homework Sheet: Recovery versus Relapse Thinking."

SUMMARY OF SESSION STEPS AND TIME MANAGEMENT

- **Step 1:** Check-in procedure (15 minutes).
- **Step 2:** Review last week's group topic, "Taking Medication" (5 minutes).
- **Step 3:** Review last week's skill practice questions on Handout 9.2, "Skill Practice Homework Sheet: Taking Medication" (5 minutes).
- **Step 4:** Distribute Handout 10.1, and discuss how changing "may as well" thinking to recovery thinking leads to recovery behaviors (30 minutes).
  - Ask members for examples of "may as well thinking.
  - Define "may as well" thinking.
  - "May as well" thinking is related to depressive thinking.
  - Fighting "may as well" thinking.
  - Learn to "hang up on your disease."
  - The central recovery rule counters "may as well" thinking.
- **Step 5:** Distribute Handout 10.2, and ask all members to practice monitoring "may as well" thinking (5 minutes).

BACKGROUND

This session reinforces the lessons that thoughts lead to behaviors—specifically, that recovery thoughts lead to recovery behaviors, and relapse thoughts lead to relapse behaviors. Therefore, learning how to recognize relapse thinking is critical to fighting these thoughts, since choosing recovery thoughts instead leads to recovery behaviors. A common type of thought logic leading to both substance use and behavior leading to mood destabilization is "may as well" thinking; for example, "I've had one drink, so I *may as well* keep drinking, since I've already blown my sobriety," or "My medication ran out yesterday and I've already missed two days of medications, so I *may as well* go the whole week without it." In this session, group members learn actively to identify "may as well" thoughts as addictive thoughts, distorted negative thoughts, or depressive thoughts, and to respond by fighting them and changing them to recovery thoughts. Group members learn that it always matters what they choose to believe, since what they choose to believe will strongly influence their behavior—for better or for worse.

Step 1: Check-in procedure (15 minutes).

Following the group leaders' announcements (e.g., expected member or leader absences, changes to the group meeting schedule or site, introductions for new members), all patients should review their weekly progress according to Handout 1.2, "Monitoring Your Symptoms: How to Check In on Your Recovery" (see Session 1). During this time, other group members are discouraged from commenting on the individual's check-in report, since relevant discussions can occur during the review of the skill practice. The group leaders should make brief summary comments that recognize and positively reinforce any thought or behavioral changes that indicate that the group members are making efforts to achieve abstinence and mood stability or to directly apply the central recovery rule. Check-in is also a time for the group leaders to listen carefully for any content that might provide a useful opportunity for the group to discuss this week's group theme; for this session, leaders will note any reports of "may as well" thinking.

Step 2: Review last week's group topic, "Taking Medication" (5 minutes).

Ask group members how they did this week considering the pros and cons of taking their medications. Ask whether they had any difficulty creating a medication log and daily calendar, and whether anyone had a better experience with taking medication this week compared to the previous week. Remind group members that people with BD ordinarily require ongoing medication treatment for good recovery and that, on the whole, taking medication produces more benefits than problems.

Step 3: Review last week's skill practice questions on Handout 9.2, "Skill Practice Homework Sheet: Taking Medication" (5 minutes).

Review last week's skill practice questions for "Taking Medication." If some group members continue to worry that their medication problems outweigh the benefits, then have the group as a whole review individual pros and cons squares in an attempt to help group members to get a different perspective. If this doesn't help, suggest that they call their prescribing clinician to discuss their concerns.

Step 4: Distribute Handout 10.1, and discuss how changing "may as well" thinking to recovery thinking leads to recovery behaviors (30 minutes).

Ask members for examples of "may as well" thinking.

Announce today's topic: "Recovery versus Relapse Thinking: It Matters What You Do." Say that the focus of this session is the idea that identifying and addressing self-defeating addictive, depressive, and manic thoughts can help group members' recovery. Write on the board, "I may as well _____." Ask the group, "Can anyone remember a time when you said to yourself, 'Well, I'm not feeling great today, so I *may as well*: (fill in the blank)?', and then doing that turned out badly?" If no one says anything, give an example, such as "I may as well turn off the alarm clock and stay in bed," or "I may as well cancel my plans to see my friend." Try to get as many participants as possible to give examples; write these on the board.

Define "may as well" thinking.

Ask the group, "Are there other phrases you might think of that say pretty much the same thing as 'may as well'?" Write group members' responses on the board; responses may include "Who cares?", "What the hell," "screw it," and "It doesn't really matter what I do." Ask the group what all of these phrases have in common. Essentially they all represent forms of negative thinking and imply that *what you decide to do doesn't make any difference.* Then ask group members whether they ever felt that way—that it really didn't matter what they chose to do.

"May as well" thinking is related to depressive thinking.

Point out that depressive thinking is often related to "may as well" thinking, in that people who become depressed may be convinced that they can't do anything to make their situation any better. You can say, "The problem with that kind of thinking, however, is that it builds on itself. For example, when you don't get out of bed or take a shower, or call someone back or eat dinner because you don't think it matters what you do, what happens?" Group members will recognize that their depression will get worse. Then say, "Yes! Things get worse instead of better. That's why depressive thinking and 'may as well' thinking are so dangerous: They both try to convince you that it doesn't matter what you do when in fact, it *always* matters what you do!"

Fighting "may as well" thinking.

"May as well" thinking occurs when addictive or depressive thinking combines with ambivalence about recovery or treatment; the patient may then conclude that the struggle for recovery simply isn't worth the effort, because things will turn out badly. As we reviewed in Session 1, "It's Two against One, but You Can Win," depressive thoughts and addictive thoughts often strengthen each other, leading to relapse. For example, depressive thoughts may make people feel that that even though they will regret their substance use the next day, escaping from their feelings for an hour or two is worth the cost. Moreover, depressive thinking can convince people that their life is going downhill anyway, so that the negative consequences of substance use don't matter. You are likely to hear people say, "When I am depressed, I can't stop myself from using." At this time, it is important to talk again about depressive thinking, which is also the subject of Session 3, "Dealing with Depression without Abusing Substances." Here, you should emphasize the "self-righteousness" and the "certainty" of depressive thinking. People who are very depressed do not *think* that their lives are going downhill; they *know* it. As mentioned in Session 3, it is often useful in discussing depressive thinking to say that being depressed is like wearing dark glasses but not being aware that you have on dark glasses. Everywhere you look, things are dark: Your past is dark, your present is dark, and your future is dark. Moreover, you think that anyone who tries to tell you that things aren't so dark merely cannot see properly, since you can see the darkness so clearly.

   After using this analogy to describe depression, you can say that the first step in dealing with depression is realizing that you have on dark glasses, so that you can take your depressive thinking with a grain of salt and understand that your pessimism is not a reflection of reality but merely a symptom of your depressive thinking. This can help to ease the burden of depressive thinking, which may in turn reduce the severity of a drug or alcohol urge.

Learn to "hang up on your disease."

After discussing depressive thinking, you can say that we are now going to talk about a skill known as "hang up on your disease." Patients may find it helpful to think about "may as well" thinking as an attempt by their depressive thoughts and addictive thoughts to gang up on them to get them to use substances. It may be useful to think of their "disease" (or diseases) as having better debating skills than their healthy side, since their unhealthy side has only one purpose (i.e., getting them to use substances), and has had much more experience than their healthy side. A useful analogy here is for group members to think of their unhealthy side as being like a telephone salesperson who calls to sell them something they don't need, which they will regret buying the next day. Starting a conversation and entering into a debate with this person plays into the salesperson's hand; they are thus likely to end up buying what the person is selling. The only way to guarantee that they do not buy anything is to *hang up the phone*. Therefore, tell them that when their depressed thoughts and their addictive thoughts say, "You may as well have just one drink; it won't matter" or "You may as well skip your medication today; one day doesn't make a difference," they should think of these thoughts as the telephone salesperson saying, "How are you tonight?" At that point, they need to escape the situation by "hanging up" on their disease and following the *central recovery rule*: "No matter what, don't drink, don't use drugs, and take your medication as prescribed—*no matter what!*"

The central recovery rule counters "may as well" thinking.

Reinforce the central recovery rule, saying,

> "This is why if you only learn the central recovery rule, you will still have learned the most important tool for your recovery. If you think to yourself, 'I may as well go on a binge because I've had a slip' (a thought process called the *abstinence violation effect*), things will get much worse for you. This is why you need to fight this kind of 'may as well' thinking by following the central recovery rule. Similarly, if you still feel depressed after taking your medication as prescribed every day, you may start thinking to yourself, 'I may as well stop taking my medication altogether, because I don't feel any better.' If you act on that thought rather than on the central recovery rule, however, you will definitely be feeling worse in a short matter of time. But if you stick to the central recovery rule, and think, 'Wait! It *matters* if I don't use now, it *matters* if I take my medication as prescribed,' then chances are good that you will head in a better direction, not worse. So **it always matters what you do!**"

With about 8–10 minutes left in the group, you should summarize two or three take-home themes that people should try to remember. You might say something like "Okay, we're near the end of today's group. Let's summarize the main points we discussed today that people should keep in mind." Encourage people to state two or three major concepts from today's session; when this is done, you should say something like

> "If you only remember two things from today's group, you should remember that when you say to yourself, 'I *may as well* do something,' you are probably about to make a bad decision; you're probably responding to depressive or addictive thinking. 'May as well' thinking can be fought with a technique called 'hang up on your disease,' and by following the central recovery rule."

You should summarize these main thoughts and write them on the whiteboard, or point them out on the bulletin board and/or the session Handout 10.1. Make sure that everybody understands these main points, then move on to the skill practice assignment.

Step 5: Distribute Handout 10.2, and ask all members to practice monitoring "may as well" thinking (5 minutes).

Review the skill practice for the next session; ask members to watch for "may as well" thinking this week, and to practice catching those thoughts and replacing them with the thought "It matters what I do." End the group session by telling group members that you look forward to seeing them again next week.

Recovery versus Relapse Thinking:
It Matters What You Do

One of the most important ideas you need to understand about recovery and relapse is that neither occurs out of the blue. Rather, a decision to abstain or to use substances, or a decision to take or not take your medication as prescribed, usually occurs as a result of certain thoughts, feelings, and behaviors. Therefore, being able to recognize and identify the thoughts that may lead to trouble can help to prevent substance use or a mood episode.

In Session 6, "Reading Your Signals: Recognizing Early Signs of Trouble," we discussed some of the early warning signs of substance use, depression, and mania, and some of the thoughts and behaviors that may precede their return. One type of thinking that all of these have in common is what can be called *"may as well" thinking*, in which you find yourself trying to choose between two very different behaviors: drinking versus sobriety, taking medication as prescribed versus not taking medication as prescribed, going to a self-help meeting versus not going, getting out of bed versus staying in bed, and so forth. If you are using "may as well" thinking, you say to yourself, "It doesn't really matter what I do. I *may as well* get high, or I may as well just stay in bed," and so forth. **"May as well" thinking, which also could be called "Who cares?" or "It doesn't matter" thinking, involves looking at two very different choices and convincing yourself (against your better judgment) that both are basically the same, so it doesn't matter which one you choose**.

Whenever you say to yourself, "I may as well . . . ," "It doesn't matter," "Who cares?" or "The hell with it," **watch out!** You may be heading for deep trouble, because you are trying to convince yourself that the choices you make in your life don't matter. This is the kind of unhealthy thinking that will lead to disaster unless you fight it! **It does matter what you do! It always matters what you do!**

When you feel that nothing that you do matters, it's because your illness is talking to you; your substance abuse, your depression, or your mania, or a combination of these illnesses is "ganging up on you" to try to bring you down. Depression and substance use can easily gang up by getting you to say to yourself, "I'm so depressed, I can't stand it. I may as well drink or take some pills, just to escape for tonight. It doesn't matter anyway." Mania can cause "may as well" thinking by getting you to think as follows: "I'm going to crash when I come down anyway, so I may as well enjoy my mania while it lasts. A little cocaine may help to make my mood even better, or alcohol may help on the way down."

"May as well" thinking is also at the center of the **abstinence violation effect**, in which people who have slipped (some people use the tern *lapsed*) may feel so badly about slipping that they keep using drugs to escape their sense of guilt ("I've blown my sobriety anyway, so I may as well really let myself go"; "It looks as if I'm heading for a manic episode anyway, so I may as well just go with the flow"; "It looks as if I'm starting to get depressed, so I may as well just let it take its course"; "I got depressed even though I was taking my medication as prescribed, so I may as well just stop my medications"). These illnesses will try to convince you to let them take you over. Don't do it! You need to fight them every step of the way! The hallmark of these disorders is a particular type of self-deception, in which they try to get you to accept the symptoms and not fight against them. By recognizing the way in which these disorders can do this, you can begin to fight back. **The most important simple message involved in fighting back is, "It matters what you do."** It matters whether you take your medication properly. It matters whether you get out of bed. It matters whether you go to a self-help meeting. It matters whether you use drugs or stay drug-free. If you have stopped your medication for 3 days, it matters whether you let it go a "little" further, or whether you restart your medications now. If you have been

(cont.)

From *Integrated Group Therapy for Bipolar Disorder and Substance Abuse* by Roger D. Weiss and Hilary Smith Connery. Copyright 2011 by The Guilford Press. Permission to photocopy this material is granted to purchasers of this book for personal use only (see copyright page for details).

using drugs for a day, it matters whether you keep using them or stop now. If you have begun spending too much money, it matters whether you stop after having spent $200 instead of $2,000. It matters because the problems you have to face will be much less serious if you catch them early, and if you fight rather than giving in to them.

One way to fight "may as well" thinking is to use a technique called "hang up on your disease." Once you realize that "may as well" thinking is a symptom of the disease of bipolar substance abuse, try to think of your disease as a telephone salesperson who calls you at home to try to sell you something you don't need. The salesperson's goal is to keep you on the phone. This person is professionally trained to do this, and the longer you stay on the phone, the more likely you are to buy something that you will later regret buying. The **only** absolutely certain way to make sure that you don't buy something you don't need (and that you will later regret) is to **hang up**. The way to "hang up on your disease" is to consistently remind yourself of the central recovery rule. Don't get into a "logical" argument on your disease's terms, because you may lose. Don't debate it. Instead, "hang up" on your disease: No matter what, don't drink, don't take drugs, and take your medication as prescribed—*no matter what*! You may wonder for a little while whether this is the best decision. You may have second thoughts. But within a short period of time, you will **know** that you have made the right decision. A return to a mood episode or substance use and all of the misery that goes with them will always be an option, but you know very well that that is not what you want. So **hang up on your disease** and stay on the road to recovery.

Remember, you are involved in a fight for control of your life. Who do you want to control your life: your healthy self or your illness? Whenever you give in to "may as well" thinking, you are letting your illness run your life. Whenever you fight that kind of thinking, **you** are running your life. And that is the way it should be.

Skill Practice Homework Sheet:
Recovery versus Relapse Thinking:
It Matters What You Do

Patient Initials: _____

Date: _____

1. Give one example of "may as well" thinking that has led you in the past into substance use.

    _____

    _____

2. List one thing you will do in the next week to fight this "may as well" thinking pattern.

    _____

    _____

3. Give one example of "may as well" thinking that has led you into an episode of mania or depression.

    _____

    _____

4. List one thing you will do in the next week to fight this "may as well" thinking pattern.

    _____

    _____

From *Integrated Group Therapy for Bipolar Disorder and Substance Abuse* by Roger D. Weiss and Hilary Smith Connery. Copyright 2011 by The Guilford Press. Permission to photocopy this material is granted to purchasers of this book for personal use only (see copyright page for details).

~~~~~~~~~~~~~~~~~~~~~~

Taking Care of Yourself

SESSION OBJECTIVES

1. Group members will be told that individuals with BD and SUD frequently don't prioritize taking proper care of themselves, and this leads to recurrence of substance use and mood episodes.

2. Group members will learn that taking care of oneself is a treatment priority and that self-care (which is healthy) is different from "being selfish" (which is unhealthy).

3. Group members will learn sleep hygiene techniques and strategies to avoid risky sexual behaviors that could lead to HIV infection, as well as other negative consequences.

MATERIALS REQUIRED

- Bulletin board with the central recovery rule, routes to recovery or relapse, and Session 11 materials posted.
- Dry erase board and markers.
- Copies of Handout 11.1, "Taking Care of Yourself."
- Copies of a list of anonymous HIV testing sites in the area.
- Copies of Handout 11.2, "Skill Practice Homework Sheet: Taking Care of Yourself."

SUMMARY OF SESSION STEPS AND TIME MANAGEMENT

- **Step 1:** Check-in procedure (15 minutes).
- **Step 2:** Review last week's group topic, "Recovery versus Relapse Thinking: It Matters What You Do" (5 minutes).
- **Step 3:** Review last week's skill practice questions on Handout 10.2, "Skill Practice Homework Sheet: Recovery versus Relapse Thinking: It Matters What You Do" (5 minutes).
- **Step 4:** Distribute Handout 11.1. Emphasize the importance of self-care for recovery, including getting a good night's sleep and avoiding HIV risk behaviors (30 minutes).
  - Discuss how group members' sleep problems relate to bipolar substance abuse.
  - Using alcohol or other substances to sleep causes poorer sleep quality and possibly addiction.
  - Sleep hygiene habits can help control bipolar disorder symptoms.
  - Remind group members that different sleep interventions work for different people.
  - Distinguish between healthy sex and unhealthy sex.
  - Define HIV infection.
  - List high-risk HIV behaviors.
  - Avoiding HIV risk behaviors using self-care skills.
- **Step 5:** Distribute Handout 11.2 and the list of local, anonymous HIV testing sites, and ask group members to pay extra attention this week to taking good care of themselves (5 minutes).

BACKGROUND

The central recovery rule is essential for self-care, but it is only the *beginning* of self-care; being fully healthy also means prioritizing a variety of healthy behaviors, such as watching one's diet, keeping up with responsibilities, and avoiding dangerous relationships and behaviors. Group members are taught to distinguish clearly between *self-care*, which refers to making healthy choices and protecting themselves from unhealthy or unsafe influences, and *selfishness*, which may involve making unhealthy choices that hurt important relationships. This session focuses on two aspects of self-care that are commonly problematic for individuals with BD and SUDs: maintaining proper sleep routines and avoiding risky sexual behavior and HIV risk behaviors. These topics are both included in one session because we have found that discussing risky sexual behaviors in the context of taking care of oneself permits group members to discuss this very sensitive subject more openly. These are important topics to discuss, because poor sleep is a common trigger for both substance use and mood destabilization. In addition, risky sexual behaviors often occur in the context of substance use or unstable mood. Reinforcing the Session 10 theme, group leaders remind members that *it always matters what people choose*, even when it may not seem important at the time.

Step 1: Check-in procedure (15 minutes).

Following the group leaders' announcements (e.g., expected member or leader absences, changes to the group meeting schedule or site, introductions for new members), all patients should review their weekly progress according to Handout 1.2, "Monitoring Your Symptoms: How to Check In on Your Recovery" (see Session 1). During this time, other group members are discouraged from commenting on the individual's check-in report, since relevant discussions can occur during the review of the skill practice. The group leaders should make brief summary comments that recognize and positively reinforce any thought or behavioral changes that indicate that the group members are making efforts to achieve abstinence and mood stability or to directly apply the central recovery rule. Check-in is also a time for the group leaders to listen carefully for any content that might provide a useful opportunity for the group to discuss this week's group theme; for this session, leaders will note any reports of sleep difficulties, or unsafe or unhealthy choices or behaviors.

Step 2: Review last week's group topic, "Recovery versus Relapse Thinking: It Matters What You Do" (5 minutes).

Ask group members whether they were able to catch themselves in the middle of "may as well" thinking, and whether they were they able to change this to "It matters what I do" thinking. Ask whether they practiced the technique "hang up on you disease." Tell members that practicing this type of thought switching is a great example of taking good care of themselves.

Step 3: Review last week's skill practice questions on Handout 10.2, "Skill Practice Homework Sheet Recovery versus Relapse Thinking: It Matters What You Do" (5 minutes).

If there are group members who found it very difficult to change their "may as well" thinking, ask other group members to help them out during the review. Remind members that being able to ask for help is another good example of taking care of themselves, and that they should not view asking others for help as "selfish" or as asking too much.

Step 4: Distribute Handout 11.1. Emphasize the importance of self-care for recovery, including getting a good night's sleep and avoiding HIV risk behaviors (30 minutes).

Announce that today's topic is "Taking Care of Yourself." Say that this session will focus on two common, problematic issues: sleep problems and risky behavior. Both of these can have a major impact on recovery and overall health.

Discuss how group members' sleep problems relate to bipolar substance abuse.

Ask the group, "How many people have had trouble with their sleep?" In general, most, if not all, of the people in the group will raise their hands. Ask group members to describe the sleep problems they have had, and write these on the board as they are reported. As you write them down, inform group members that many types of sleep disturbance may be related to either BD or substance use. For example, if a member describes early morning awakening, you may note that this is a typical symptom of depression; if a member describes not sleeping but still feeling energetic or "hyper," you may note that this pattern is typical of mania or hypomania. Also mention that many substances of abuse and some medications can have side effects that alter sleep by either keeping people awake or causing them to sleep too much.

Using alcohol or other substances to sleep causes poorer sleep quality and possibly addiction.

Now ask the group, "Has anyone ever used alcohol or other substances because they couldn't sleep?" This is a common occurrence, but it is a dangerous strategy for fixing sleep disturbances. Explain to the group that alcohol and benzodiazepine sedatives (e.g., clonazepam [Klonopin], lorazepam [Ativan], diazepam [Valium], and alprazolam [Xanax] may temporarily improve sleep but likely decrease the quality of sleep over time, so that the sleep problem gets worse and more of the substance is required to fall asleep. This vicious cycle can be the beginning of an addiction problem. Note that it is always dangerous to "be your own doctor," and part of taking good care of yourself includes asking your doctor or nurse for help if you are having trouble with sleep.

Substance use can cause a variety of types of sleep problems, depending on the drugs used and the pattern of use. Some drugs, such as cocaine or amphetamine, can cause difficulty falling asleep and poor sleep quality during periods of active use, followed by too much sleep after stopping use. Alcohol may initially help people to sleep but can produce poor sleep quality, with frequent awakenings during the night and a sense of not feeling rested in the morning. People who have been dependent on opioids (narcotics) or benzodiazepines often have severe difficulty falling asleep after stopping these drugs; this problem can last for a very long time—from weeks to months.

Sleep hygiene habits can help control bipolar disorder symptoms.

Next, tell the group:

> "Getting at least 7 hours of quality sleep is one of the best natural "medications" for keeping the symptoms of bipolar disorder controlled. The opposite is also true: not having a healthy sleep pattern is one of the most common triggers for having a mood episode. There are strategies that you can learn, listed in Handout 11.1, to improve your sleep patterns and quality of sleep. We call these strategies *sleep hygiene*, because they are core skills for taking care of yourself, similar to showering and brushing your teeth daily. Let's go over these sleep hygiene strategies together."

The handout lists the following 10 effective sleep hygiene strategies:

1. Monitor your sleep with a daily calendar or log.
2. Set a regular time to go to bed and to wake up *every* day of the week, even on weekends.

3. Avoid caffeine, particularly after 12:00 noon.
4. Exercise during the day, but avoid strenuous exercise in the evening.
5. Don't watch TV or use the computer just before bedtime.
6. If you cannot fall asleep, don't lie in bed awake, tossing and turning. Rather, get up, get out of bed, and do something quiet, such as reading a book that is likely to make you sleepy. Don't watch TV or do something physically active; those are likely to wake you up even more.
7. Avoid "clock watching" in the middle of the night, which tends to make you more worried about not sleeping. Therefore, turn the clock away from you at night.
8. Don't stay in bed in the morning. Instead, get up.
9. Don't nap for more than 20 minutes during the day.
10. If sleep problems continue, ask your therapist or prescribing clinician for help.

Remind group members that different sleep interventions work for different people.

One problem you may have during this part of the session is that some group members have tried a variety of interventions for sleep problems, with very little success. It is important to remain upbeat about this issue, even though some people in the group may have chronic sleep disorders that may be refractory to these and many other strategies. In such a case, talk about the fact that there are a number of different interventions for sleep problems, and different people respond to different interventions. If some group members are genuinely struggling with chronic insomnia in spite of taking good care of themselves, you may want to suggest that they consult with their doctor about obtaining a sleep study with a specialist.

Distinguish between healthy sex and unhealthy sex.

Begin the group discussion on risky sexual behavior with a sense of humor; you might say, "Sleep specialists say that you should never use the bed for other activities, such as watching TV or using the computer or reading, because these will interfere with sound sleep. They say the bed should be used only for sleep and for sex. We've talked about sleep. Now we can talk about sex." Go to the board and write two columns titled "healthy sex" and "unhealthy sex," and ask group members to suggest examples for each column. Examples of healthy sex might include proper use of barrier (condom) contraceptives, having sex with someone you know very well and can trust, and being sober when you have sex. Examples of unhealthy sex might include not using barrier contraception, having sex with people you barely know, having sex with multiple partners, having sex while you are drunk or high, having risky sex because you are manic, having sex with someone who may hurt you, or having sex to "pay for" drugs. Then ask the group,

"If you look at these two columns, you might notice that there is a difference between healthy sex and unhealthy sex, like when we looked at the difference between taking care of yourself and being selfish. Let's ask the same questions we did earlier about these examples: What are the motives for each? What would be the likely impact on the other person? On yourself?"

This is to generate group discussion that avoiding risky sexual behaviors involves the same skills as other self-care topics: thinking it through, staying sober, and making good choices about what is beneficial to your health.

Define HIV infection.

Now ask, "Who here can tell the group about HIV infection?" Elicit a description, or provide one yourself (*human immunodeficiency virus*, a potentially deadly disease that can be passed from person to person by unprotected sex and by needle sharing).

List high-risk HIV behaviors.

Ask the group for examples of poor choices that would put a person at risk for contracting HIV, and write these on the board. These are listed in Handout 11.1:

- Sharing paraphernalia such as needles during injection drug use.
- Engaging in risky sexual behaviors.
  - Having sex without a condom.
  - Having sex with multiple partners.
  - Having sex with someone you barely know.
  - Having sex with someone you think may be HIV positive.
  - Having sex when you are drunk, high, or manic (and less likely to protect yourself, such as with proper condom use).

Common triggers for making unhealthy choices include being intoxicated, lonely, bored, depressed, manic, or impulsive. Note also that "may as well" thinking can lead to risky sexual behaviors (e.g., "I may as well have sex with this person. Who cares if he/she is HIV positive? My life can't get any worse than it already is").

Avoiding HIV risk behaviors using self-care skills.

Tell the group:

> "I'm sure that some of you have engaged in a variety of risky behaviors. It might have involved driving too fast, having sex with the wrong person, or maybe sharing needles. I'm sure there are other times when the temptation to do these things has come up, and you've resisted. What have been the circumstances in which you have been able to resist that temptation, and what's been going on when you haven't?"

Allow the group to review self-care, making healthy choices, and fighting the thoughts or feelings that often lead to making unhealthy or unsafe choices; this puts HIV risk behaviors into the context of other self-care strategies discussed throughout the group treatment. Finally, tell group members that they should never worry alone if they think they have been in a high-risk situation for contracting HIV, and refer them to the list of local, anonymous HIV testing sites available.

With about 8–10 minutes left in the group, you should summarize two or three take-home themes that people should try to remember. You might say something like "Okay, we're near the end of today's group. Let's summarize the main points we discussed today that people should keep in mind." Encourage people to state two or three major concepts from today's session; when this is done, say something like "If you only remember a few things from today's group, you should remember the following: Taking good care of yourself is important for your recovery and your overall health; this includes practicing good sleep hygiene and avoiding risky behavior. You should summarize these main thoughts and write them on the whiteboard, or point them out on the bulletin board and/or session Handout 11.1. Make sure that everybody understands these main points, then move on to the skill practice assignment.

Step 5: Distribute Handout 11.2 and the list of local, anonymous HIV testing sites, and ask group members to pay extra attention this week to taking good care of themselves (5 minutes).

Pass out the skill practice and a list of anonymous HIV testing sites in your local area. Let group members know that these sites can serve as an excellent resource if they are ever concerned about their HIV risk. Tell them that you look forward to seeing them again next week.

Taking Care of Yourself

A common problem for people with bipolar disorder and substance abuse is that they don't always take good care of themselves. **Taking good care of yourself means that you make it a priority to make healthy choices and stick with the central recovery rule** ("No matter what, don't drink, don't use drugs, and take your medication as prescribed—no matter what!"). Taking care of yourself doesn't mean you are being selfish or that you care only about yourself. It means you understand that if you don't take care of yourself, not only will you be unhappy, but you will also make people you care about unhappy. This handout will help you to make good decisions about two important health issues: getting a good night's sleep, and avoiding risky sexual behaviors that may put you at risk for HIV infection, as well as other sexually transmitted diseases.

SLEEP

Sleep problems are very common among people with bipolar disorder and substance use disorders. A change in your usual sleep pattern is often one of the earliest signs that you may be beginning a mood episode. For example, waking up early in the morning may be an early warning sign of depression; feeling as if you don't need sleep may be the first sign of hypomania or mania. People often notice changes in their sleep routines before they experience other symptoms, so monitoring sleep patterns can be an excellent way of picking up on early signs of mood problems.

Poor sleep patterns may be a trigger for substance use as well, since people who can't fall asleep may resort to drinking alcohol or misusing sleep medications. Unfortunately, using alcohol or sleep medications to fall asleep often decreases "deep sleep" and leads to waking up in the middle of the night, which makes the problem worse instead of better. Drinking and misusing sleep medicines may also worsen symptoms of bipolar disorder, which can worsen sleep problems. Of course, misusing alcohol and sleep medicines can also lead to being addicted to them, which only adds another problem to your life.

WHAT IS "SLEEP HYGIENE"?

Sleep hygiene is a term used to describe healthy habits that promote good sleep. Here are 10 effective sleep hygiene strategies:

1. Monitor your sleep with a daily calendar or log.

Keeping a simple log of your sleep patterns: write down every day when you get to sleep, how long you slept (or didn't because you found yourself tossing and turning through the night), and when you wake up. This is your easiest strategy for detecting changes in your sleep early on. It is also very helpful to bring a sleep log with you to appointments with your prescribing doctor or nurse.

2. Set a regular time to go to bed and to wake up *every* day of the week, even on weekends.

This is critical! You might think that this is "boring," but when it comes to natural "medications" to control symptoms of bipolar disorder, this one is the most effective methods.

(cont.)

From *Integrated Group Therapy for Bipolar Disorder and Substance Abuse* by Roger D. Weiss and Hilary Smith Connery. Copyright 2011 by The Guilford Press. Permission to photocopy this material is granted to purchasers of this book for personal use only (see copyright page for details).

3. Avoid caffeine, particularly after 12:00 noon.

With the availability of supersize coffees and "energy" drinks, this may seem difficult, but you need to know that caffeine is your enemy if it is not taken in small, morning doses. Not only will it disrupt your sleep cycle (a trigger for both mood episodes and substance use), but if you are prone to anxiety, it can make that worse as well.

4. Exercise during the day, but avoid strenuous exercise in the evening.

Exercise is great for sleep: it enhances "deeper" stages of sleep that really restore you. But exercising at night is a problem, because it can wake you up so much that you will have difficulty falling asleep. Avoid exercising in the evening.

5. Don't watch TV or use the computer just before bedtime.

The visual stimulation of TV and computer screens will make it harder for you to fall asleep when you wish. Many people make the mistake of "falling asleep with the TV on for white noise"; this is a terrible thing for sleep because it keeps you in "lighter" stages of sleep that lead to a restless night. If your favorite show is on late at night, investigate options for recording your show, so that you can watch it during daytime hours.

6. If you cannot fall asleep, don't lie in bed awake, tossing and turning.

This is a common mistake. If you can't fall asleep for 15 minutes longer than it usually takes, get out of bed, sit up, and try reading. **Do not stay in bed for a long time if you can't fall asleep!** You should establish bed as a place where you sleep, not a place where you toss, turn, and worry about not sleeping. Similarly, do not spend time resting in bed during the day. If you need to rest, do it somewhere else.

7. Avoid "clock watching" in the middle of the night, which tends to make you more worried about not sleeping.

Clock watching only builds up anxiety and makes it more difficult to sleep. If you need to wake up at a certain hour in the morning, set your alarm, but turn the clock away from you.

8. Don't stay in bed in the morning. Instead, get up.

Staying in bed during the daytime only worsens sleep patterns. Fight the temptation to sleep during the day. Get up and get active, even if you don't feel like it.

9. Don't nap for more than 20 minutes during the day.

Research has shown that after a 15- to 20-minute nap, people wake up more refreshed. A nap that is longer than 20 minutes tends to drain energy and will make you sleepier when you wake up than you were before you took the nap.

10. If sleep problems continue, ask your therapist or prescribing clinician for help.

Talking about your sleep patterns and potentially adjusting your medication may help you to improve your sleep, which will improve your mood and reduce your likelihood of substance use. If you keep having problems with sleep despite good sleep hygiene habits and stable medications, you may need to consult a sleep specialist or schedule a sleep study to find out the cause of your sleep problems.

(cont.)

AVOIDING RISKY SEXUAL BEHAVIOR AND HIV RISK BEHAVIORS

Having bipolar disorder and substance use disorders can increase a person's risk to have unhealthy or unsafe sexual behaviors that increase the risk of sexually transmitted diseases, such as HIV (human immunodeficiency virus: a deadly disease), hepatitis B and C, gonorrhea, chlamydia, and herpes. Risky sexual behaviors also increase the chances of having an unintended pregnancy.

High-risk behaviors that can lead to unhealthy choices about sexual behavior:

- Sharing paraphernalia ("works") such as needles during injection drug use.
- Engaging in risky sexual behaviors.
  - Having sex without a condom.
  - Having sex with multiple partners.
  - Having sex with someone you barely know.
  - Having sex with someone you think may be HIV positive.
  - Having sex when you are drunk, high, or manic (and less likely to protect yourself, such as with proper condom use).

The best way to reduce HIV risk is to follow your treatment program. Follow the central recovery rule (abstain from alcohol and drugs and take your medication as prescribed), hang around with people you know to be safe and responsible, and attend whatever therapy is being recommended.

As many people are aware, the major risk factor for HIV infection is an exchange of bodily fluids, which typically occurs during (1) sexual activity, or (2) sharing of drug use paraphernalia, especially needles. The proper use of latex condoms can reduce (but not eliminate) the risk of sexually transmitted HIV infection. If you relapse to needle use (and we certainly hope that you don't), you should always use a clean, sterile needle from a pharmacy or a needle-exchange program. Keep in mind that **any substance use increases the risk that you will make an unhealthy choice about needle sharing or sexual behavior**, so follow the central recovery rule!

HIV testing can determine whether you have been infected with HIV, the virus that causes AIDS. It is important to note, however, that it may take up to 6 months after your last exposure to test positive for HIV infection. Therefore, if you have an HIV test that comes out negative, you should be tested again 6 months after your last exposure to be sure you have not contracted HIV. Anonymous, free testing services are widely available, where you can receive HIV testing. **Don't worry alone! Ask for help. That is one of the best ways you can take good care of yourself**.

Skill Practice Homework Sheet:
Taking Care of Yourself

Patient Initials: _____

Date: _____

1. List one way you are currently taking good care of yourself.

   _____

   _____

   _____

2. List one new thing that you will do in the upcoming week to help you take better care of yourself.

   _____

   _____

   _____

3. Name something that you do, or will start to do, for healthier sleep.

   _____

   _____

   _____

4. Name one behavior that protects you from getting HIV.

   _____

   _____

   _____

From *Integrated Group Therapy for Bipolar Disorder and Substance Abuse* by Roger D. Weiss and Hilary Smith Connery. Copyright 2011 by The Guilford Press. Permission to photocopy this material is granted to purchasers of this book for personal use only (see copyright page for details).

SESSION 12

Ⓒ〰〰〰〰〰〰〰〰〰Ⓓ

Taking the Group with You

SESSION OBJECTIVES

1. Group members will review the central recovery rule and discuss how they have applied this rule to support their recovery from BD and SUD.
2. Group members will review the highlights of the preceding group session topics and identify the skills that have worked best for their recovery. Group leaders will emphasize the importance of reviewing all the session handouts on a regular basis.
3. Group members will list recovery supports they have developed outside the group and discuss how these are important to maintaining mood stability and sobriety.

MATERIALS REQUIRED

- Bulletin board with the central recovery rule, routes to recovery or relapse, and Session 12 materials posted.
- Dry erase board and markers.
- Copies of Handout 12.1, "Taking the Group with You."
- Copies of Handout 12.2, "Skill Practice Homework Sheet: Taking the Group with You."

SUMMARY OF SESSION STEPS AND TIME MANAGEMENT

- **Step 1:** Check-in procedure (15 minutes).
- **Step 2:** Review last week's group topic, "Taking Care of Yourself" (5 minutes).

- **Step 3:** Review last week's skill practice questions on Handout 11.2, "Skill Practice Homework Sheet: Taking Care of Yourself" (5 minutes).

- **Step 4:** Distribute Handout 12.1, and review the central recovery rule and other main lessons of the IGT sessions (30 minutes).

- **Step 5:** Distribute Handout 12.2, and ask members to think about being grateful to people who have helped them in their recovery (5 minutes).

BACKGROUND

As originally designed, this session is meant to be a termination session in a "closed" group (i.e., a group in which everyone begins and ends the group treatment at the same time). If you are running your group in a closed fashion, then this group session is appropriate as a final group. However, many people run IGT as an "open" group, in which patients may enter or leave at any time. If a patient wants to stay for more than 12 weeks, then some topics will be repeated; those patients who leave before completing 12 sessions will not review all of the topics. Therefore, this particular group session may be postponed if many of the members have just recently entered an open group. If several members have been in the group for 6 weeks or more, however, this group can serve as an excellent review to help group members think through ways they will be able to use the group over time.

This session is designed to promote group members' self-efficacy for maintaining the skills they have developed throughout their participation in IGT. The central recovery rule is reviewed, along with the main lessons of preceding groups. Routine review of session handouts is recommended to maintain recovery skills. Group leaders encourage members to focus on utilizing the skills that members (and their recovery supports) believe to be most effective for them individually, and discuss the ways recovery supports outside the group have been, and will continue to be, an essential part of each member's recovery process.

Step 1: Check-in procedure (15 minutes).

Following the group leaders' announcements (e.g., expected member or leader absences, changes to the group meeting schedule or site, introductions for new members), all patients should review their weekly progress according to Handout 1.2, "Monitoring Your Symptoms: How to Check In on Your Recovery" (see Session 1). During this time, other group members are discouraged from commenting on the individual's check-in report, since relevant discussions can occur during the review of the skill practice. The group leaders should make brief summary comments that recognize and positively reinforce any thought or behavioral changes that indicate that the group members are making efforts to achieve abstinence and mood stability or to directly apply the central recovery rule. Check-in is also a time for the group leaders to listen carefully for any content that might provide a useful opportunity for the group to discuss this week's group theme; for this session, leaders will highlight individual ways of applying recovery skills and of using social supports outside the group to promote recovery.

Step 2: Review last week's group topic, "Taking Care of Yourself" (5 minutes).

Ask group members how they did this week with trying new things to take better care of themselves, and inquire as to whether this effort made a difference. Ask if anyone tried the sleep hygiene methods discussed the previous week, and how they worked out. Remind members that all people with BD should consider sleep hygiene as another "medicine" to help their mood and their substance abuse problem.

Step 3: Review last week's skill practice questions on Handout 11.2, "Skill Practice Homework Sheet: Taking Care of Yourself" (5 minutes).

If some members are not taking good care of themselves, ask the group to help those members to think of reasons why they might benefit from taking better care of themselves.

Step 4: Distribute Handout 12.1, and review the central recovery rule and other main lessons of the integrated group therapy sessions (30 minutes).

Announce today's topic: "Taking the Group With You." The way you summarize this group will depend on the circumstances described earlier, namely, whether or not a significant number of people are leaving the group. If so, you can say, "A number of you are leaving the group after today, and that is always a good opportunity to step back and see what has been particularly helpful for people in the group." If very few people are leaving, or if no one is leaving but most people have been in the group for 6 weeks or more, you might say, "Every once in a while, it's a good idea to step back and review the various topics we have talked about in the group to see how things are going and how people are using the tools they've learned here to help their recovery." If there are few experienced group members and few people leaving, then this particular group session may be skipped and another session substituted, depending on the specific issues that group members are facing.

Ask the group members, "What have you found helpful about this group so far?" Write down the skills or ideas that members report to be most helpful. As you write these down, ask, "Do other people find this helpful as well?" You may use this list to review the main teaching points of the preceding group sessions, which are summarized in the session handout as follows:

1. *Central recovery rule* ("No matter what, don't drink, don't use drugs, and take your medication as prescribed every day—no matter what!").
2. "AAA method" for managing triggers (*avoid* triggers where possible, don't face triggers *alone*, distract from triggers by getting *active* or getting *away* from them).
3. Fight depressive thinking with recovery thinking.
4. Try to see things from the other person's view to develop healthy relationships.
5. Work on acceptance of your illnesses and focus on taking care of yourself.
6. Know your early warning signs and ask for help early on.
7. Practice saying "no" to drugs and alcohol; use snapshot versus video thinking.
8. Use self-help groups to support your recovery.
9. Take your medication as prescribed every day.

10. Choose recovery thinking over relapse thinking; "hang up on your disease."
11. Take care of yourself (by practicing sleep hygiene and avoiding risky sexual behaviors).

As you review the main lessons, ask group members, "Who helps you the most with this?" Common answers will include family members, friends, sponsors, other members of self-help groups, and treating clinicians. Emphasize that recovery is hard work and should not be fought alone; learning to ask for help is an essential part of the recovery process.

With about 8–10 minutes left in the group, you should summarize two or three take-home themes that people should try to remember. You might say something like "Okay, we're near the end of today's session. Let's summarize the main points we discussed today that people should keep in mind." Encourage people to state two or three major concepts from today's session; when this is done, you should say something like "If you only remember a few things from today's session, you should remember the following: that you should use the tools from this group that are most helpful to you and continue to review what you've learned here, since recovery is a lifelong process." Summarize these main thoughts and write them on the whiteboard, or point them out on the bulletin board and/or the session topic handout. Make sure that everybody understands these main points, then move on to the skill practice assignment.

Step 5: Distribute Handout 12.2, and ask members to think about being grateful to people who have helped them in their recovery (5 minutes).

If there are members leaving the group, remind them to follow the central recovery rule, to review their session handouts regularly, and to keep up with people or self-help groups that support their recovery, since recovery is a lifelong process. Tell the rest of the group members that you look forward to seeing them again next week.

HANDOUT 12.1

Taking the Group with You

Below is a summary of the main ideas from earlier group sessions:

1. **Central recovery rule** ("No matter what, don't drink, don't use drugs, and take your medication as prescribed—no matter what!").
2. **AAA method** for managing triggers (*Avoid* triggers when possible. Don't face triggers *alone*. Distract yourself from triggers by getting *active* or getting *away*.)
3. **Fight depressive thinking** with recovery thinking.
4. **Try to see things from the other person's view** to develop healthy relationships.
5. **Work on acceptance** of your illnesses and focus on taking care of yourself.
6. **Know your early warning signs** and ask for help early on.
7. **Practice saying "no" to drugs and alcohol**; use snapshot versus video thinking.
8. **Use self-help groups** to support your recovery.
9. **Take your medication as prescribed** every day.
10. **Choose recovery thinking** over relapse thinking; "hang up on your disease."
11. **Take care of yourself** (by practicing sleep hygiene and avoiding risky sexual behaviors).

You may remember some of these ideas better than others, and some will work better for you than others. It is important to review your session handouts regularly to remind yourself about the recovery skills you have learned during the group sessions and to keep your skills fresh. Here are some other suggestions for keeping up your recovery between groups.

Build up other supports.

People who have done well have generally built up other supports during the group sessions that have helped them between sessions and after they finished the group. Attending this group is a bit like taking a course in school. When you have finished the course, you may know the material well, but if you don't use it every day and "live" it, you will eventually forget what you have learned. Without practice, and without the continued use of the recovery tools discussed in this group, the thinking and behavior patterns that have been encouraged in this group will soon be forgotten. People who have done well after ending this group have generally done some or all of the following:

- Continued to discuss helpful ideas from the group with their case manager or therapist, doctor or nurse, sponsor, and family or friends
- Continued to ask for help and feedback from their case manager or therapist, doctor or nurse, sponsor, and family or friends
- Entered a therapy group
- Entered or continued with individual therapy
- Attended self-help groups (AA, NA, SMART Recovery, Dual Recovery, Double Trouble, or Depression and Bipolar Support Alliance [DBSA])
- Continued to offer and receive support from other members of the group

(cont.)

From *Integrated Group Therapy for Bipolar Disorder and Substance Abuse* by Roger D. Weiss and Hilary Smith Connery. Copyright 2011 by The Guilford Press. Permission to photocopy this material is granted to purchasers of this book for personal use only (see copyright page for details).

Review and continue to review session handouts.

People who have used this group successfully in the past have latched onto certain key ideas or phrases such as "no matter what," "the AAA method," or "may as well" thinking. Keeping some of these ideas in mind has helped them either to avoid trouble or to cope with high-risk situations. The longer you are away from the group, the more likely you are to forget some of the key ideas of the group unless you review them. Remember, unlike in school, there is no final exam at the end of this group. Instead, you will be tested for the rest of your life. It is therefore a good idea to reread at least one session handout every week.

Identify the recovery thoughts and recovery plans that work well for you.

One of the major ideas behind this group is to present many different recovery thoughts and behaviors, and to realize that some ideas will be very helpful to certain people and less helpful to others. If enough recovery thoughts and behaviors are presented, most people who attend this group will find some of them helpful. Therefore, focus on using the skills and thoughts that you find most useful. If the **central recovery rule** ("No matter what") is helpful to you, use it over and over again, so that it becomes automatic. If you find the **AAA method** helpful, use it. If particular ideas don't work very well for you, try them out for a while, but don't be discouraged. If another approach helps you to get through difficult situations, use that instead. No one will remember all of the material in all of these group sessions, but if you can remember a few key phrases and a few central ideas, you will be able to use them to continue your recovery.

Prepare yourself for active recovery between groups and after the group.

Everyone gets something different from the group: (1) support from other group members; (2) a place to talk about bipolar disorder and substance abuse at the same time; (3) a chance to see how other people have dealt with situations similar to those you are facing; (4) information about recovery; and (5) the peer pressure and support of having to report each week at the check-in. Begin now to develop a plan to replace those parts of the group that you find most helpful, so that you can use them in your recovery between sessions or when you no longer participate in the group.

Summary

By taking the most helpful aspects of the group with you, you will be able to achieve positive recovery outside of group participation. Never forget that "It matters what you do," and keep the central recovery rule in mind:

"No matter what, don't drink, don't use drugs, and take your medication as prescribed—no matter what!"

Skill Practice Homework Sheet:
Taking the Group with You

Patient Initials: _____

Date: _____

1. Please write down what you have found most helpful about this group.

    _____

    _____

    _____

    _____

    _____

    _____

2. Please write down how you will maintain that when you are no longer in the group.

    _____

    _____

    _____

    _____

    _____

    _____

    _____

    _____

From *Integrated Group Therapy for Bipolar Disorder and Substance Abuse* by Roger D. Weiss and Hilary Smith Connery. Copyright 2011 by The Guilford Press. Permission to photocopy this material is granted to purchasers of this book for personal use only (see copyright page for details).

APPENDIX A

(OOOOOOOOOOOOOOOOOOO)

Rating Adherence and Fidelity

Ensuring That Integrated Group Therapy Is Done Properly

When you initially implement IGT in your own practice, it can be helpful to have a checklist of core features of IGT to ensure that you are performing IGT properly. Similarly, if you run a substance abuse treatment program or a mental health clinic in which IGT is being introduced, you may want to observe the clinicians working in your agency as they conduct IGT groups. One tool that we have used to evaluate and improve therapist performance through supervision is the Integrated Group Therapy Therapist Adherence Rating Form. This checklist allows therapists to review their performance themselves, to see whether they included the key elements of IGT. Moreover, it enables supervisors to observe IGT groups or review taped sessions and evaluate the degree to which the therapist conducted the group according to the core principles of IGT.

The rating form is accompanied by a guideline for scoring the form. Each element of the group is rated on a 0 to 4-point scale, in which a score of 4 represents *full adherence* to the core principles of IGT, a score of 2 is considered *adequate adherence*, and a score of 0 represents a *complete lack of adherence* to IGT principles. It is important to recognize that this rating sheet is only a guideline, not a hard-and-fast set of rules; therapists need both to balance the desirability of adhering to the core principles of IGT and to respond to the issues that group members raise. Therefore, if a group member says in the check-in that her mother died during the past week, the therapist may decide to depart somewhat from the planned session outline in order to respond sensitively to that group member's acute distress. Deviating from the session outline should be done judiciously and infrequently, however, since group members will often be dealing with difficult issues in their lives that could derail the focus of IGT. As with all aspects of conducting IGT groups, using good clinical judgment is always the first principle of successful treatment.

Integrated Group Therapy Therapist Adherence Rating Form

Rater: _____

Therapist: _____

Date: _____

Session Topic: _____

INSTRUCTIONS FOR RATER

Please indicate in the left column ("adherence") the degree to which the therapist engaged in the described behavior. Please rate the quality ("competence") of the behavior in the right column. Please note that a competence rating takes into account whether or not a therapist *should* have performed this action. Thus, if the therapist does *not* do something that you believe he or she *should* have done, the competence score will be *low*. However, if the therapist does *not* do something that you believe should *not* have been done, then the competence rating will be *high*. Please use the "Guidelines for Completing the Therapist Evaluation Form" in determining your scores.

0	1	2	3	4
Not at all	Slightly	Somewhat	Considerably	To a great degree

THERAPEUTIC SKILL/TASK

Adherence	Competence	
Score (0–4)		

General Group Therapy Skills

_____ _____   1. Made the didactic presentation lively and engaging.

_____ _____   2. Encouraged patients to openly discuss their feelings and experiences.

_____ _____   3. Created an atmosphere of trust, respect, and confidentiality.

_____ _____   4. Was attentive to cues.

Skills Specific to Integrated Group Therapy

_____ _____   5. Focused primarily on current issues as opposed to childhood issues.

_____ _____   6. Stressed a cognitive-behavioral model.

_____ _____   7. Presented a core theme.

_____ _____   8. Completed check-in for each patient (reviewed substance use, overall mood for the week, medication adherence, high-risk situations, coping skills, skill practice; limited check-in to 15 minutes).

_____ _____   9. Displayed mastery of didactic material.

(cont.)

From *Integrated Group Therapy for Bipolar Disorder and Substance Abuse* by Roger D. Weiss and Hilary Smith Connery. Copyright 2011 by The Guilford Press. Permission to photocopy this material is granted to purchasers of this book for personal use only (see copyright page for details).

_____	_____	10. Focused on the effects of bipolar disorder and substance use disorder on each other.
_____	_____	11. Focused on the similarities between bipolar disorder and substance use disorder.
_____	_____	12. Stressed the importance of medication adherence.
_____	_____	13. Stressed the importance of abstinence.
_____	_____	14. Balanced the didactic and discussion parts of the session.
_____	_____	15. Overall Performance Rating

Guidelines for Completing the Therapist Adherence Rating Form for Integrated Group Therapy

General Group Therapy Skills

1. *Made the didactic presentation lively and engaging.*

   Adherence Rating

   0 The therapist presented the didactic material in an unengaging and boring manner, with little apparent interest in the topic or the task at hand.

   2 There were times when the therapist appeared interested and sparked the interest of the patients, and other times when the therapist was unengaging.

   4 The therapist clearly demonstrated interest in the topic and in engaging the group, and geared the presentation in such a way as to be maximally engaging.

2. *Encouraged patients to discuss their feelings and experiences openly.*

   Adherence Rating

   0 The therapist cut patients off frequently; actively discouraged expressions of affect.

   2 The therapist allowed patients to express affects and to discuss their experiences, but did not elicit feedback very much. The therapist did not actively cut patients off unless they were manic.

   4 The therapist regularly encouraged patients to discuss their feelings and experiences, and elicited feedback regularly.

3. *Created an atmosphere of trust, respect, and confidentiality.*

   Adherence Rating

   0 The therapist created a disrespectful atmosphere, allowing patients to criticize each other without therapist intervention, to engage in power struggles, and to scapegoat each other.

   2 The therapist did a reasonably good job of creating a respectful and trustful atmosphere.

   4 The therapist did an excellent job, creating an atmosphere of trust and respect, encouraging constructive and respectful feedback among patients, and offering suggestions to patients in a highly respectful manner.

4. *Was attentive to cues.*

   Adherence Rating

   0 The therapist ignored important obvious and subtle (i.e., verbal and nonverbal) cues.

   2 The therapist was attentive to obvious cues and somewhat attentive to subtle cues.

   4 The therapist was extremely attentive to important obvious and subtle cues.

Skills Specific to Integrated Group Therapy

5. *Focused primarily on current issues as opposed to childhood issues.*

   Adherence Rating

   0 The therapist focused primarily on childhood issues, taking current issues and putting them in the context of childhood issues.

   (cont.)

From *Integrated Group Therapy for Bipolar Disorder and Substance Abuse* by Roger D. Weiss and Hilary Smith Connery. Copyright 2011 by The Guilford Press. Permission to photocopy this material is granted to purchasers of this book for personal use only (see copyright page for details).

2   The therapist focused approximately evenly on current issues and childhood issues.

4   The therapist did not attend to patients' childhood experiences at all; focused only on the present and future.

6. *Stressed a cognitive-behavioral model.*

   Adherence Rating

   0   The therapist ignored important opportunities to ask patients about underlying thoughts or relate behaviors to underlying thoughts.

   2   The therapist asked about underlying thoughts or brought them to the group's attention approximately half of the time when there was a good opportunity to do so.

   4   The therapist regularly related underlying cognitions to patients' problematic behaviors.

7. *Presented a core theme.*

   Adherence Rating

   0   The therapist made no effort to present a core theme to the group.

   2   While the therapist presented a core theme, the patients were only partially able to pick up on it.

   4   A core theme was clearly articulated by the therapist and understood by the patients.

8. *Completed check-in for each patient (reviewed substance use, overall mood for the week, medication adherence, high-risk situations, coping skills, skill practice; limited check-in to 15 minutes).*

   Adherence Rating

   0   The therapist violated at least three of the preceding components (e.g., surpassed the 15-minute limit; omitted having a patient who was present check in; let a patient omit substance use).

   2   The therapist completed three of the check-in components listed earlier.

   4   The therapist completed all of the check-in components for every patient present at the check-in.

9. *Displayed mastery of didactic material.*

   Adherence Rating

   0   The therapist seemed confused and disorganized about the didactic material presented.

   2   The therapist was moderately knowledgeable about the didactic material but showed some areas of weakness.

   4   The therapist showed a clear and accurate understanding of the factual material presented in the didactic portion of the session.

10. *Focused on the effects of bipolar disorder and substance use disorder on each other.*

   Adherence Rating

   0   The therapist ignored obvious opportunities to bring up the effects of the two disorders on each other.

   2   The therapist addressed the effects of the disorders on each other in a reasonable but relatively simple way.

   4   The therapist was highly attentive to the effects of the two disorders on each other, drawing patients' attention to the topic.

(cont.)

173

11. *Focused on the similarities between bipolar disorder and substance use disorder.*

    Adherence Rating

    0   The therapist ignored obvious opportunities to bring up similarities between the two disorders.

    2   The therapist addressed the similarities between the two disorders in a reasonable but relatively simple way.

    4   The therapist was highly attentive to the similarities between the two disorders, drawing patients' attention to the topic.

12. *Stressed the importance of medication adherence.*

    Adherence Rating

    0   The therapist ignored the issue of medication adherence despite opportunities to bring it up.

    2   The therapist occasionally brought up issues relating to medication adherence but missed some opportunities to do so and did not discuss the importance of medication adherence.

    4   The therapist asked excellent questions about medication adherence issues, then followed up with appropriate responses and interventions, stressing the importance of medication adherence.

13. *Stressed the importance of abstinence.*

    Adherence Rating

    0   The therapist ignored substance use, urges, upcoming risks for use, or the need to abstain.

    2   The therapist occasionally brought up issues about substance use, urges, and upcoming risks for use but missed some opportunities to do so, and did not discuss the importance of abstinence.

    4   The therapist asked excellent questions about substance use, urges, and upcoming risks, then followed up with appropriate responses and interventions, stressing the importance of abstinence.

14. *Balanced the didactic and discussion parts of the session.*

    Adherence Rating

    0   The therapist allowed the discussion to wander aimlessly, with no relevance to the didactic material presented.

    2   The therapist was somewhat able to blend the didactic material with a discussion session, although there were some awkward spots.

    4   The therapist blended the didactic and the discussion session skillfully, so that the new information presented in the didactic session blended well with patients' experiences.

15. *Overall Performance Rating.*

    0   This session did not conform even slightly to general principles of integrated group therapy.

    2   There were aspects of conformity to overall principles of integrated group therapy, but the therapist missed obvious opportunities to integrate the treatment of the two disorders.

    4   The treatment was well-integrated, and the key principles of integrated group therapy were followed.

Bulletin Board Material

From *Integrated Group Therapy for Bipolar Disorder and Substance Abuse* by Roger D. Weiss and Hilary Smith Connery. Copyright 2011 by The Guilford Press. Permission to photocopy this material is granted to purchasers of this book for personal use only (see copyright page for details).

Session-Specific Bulletin Board Material

It's Two against One, but You Can Win!

- Two opponents—they are on the same team.
- Battle against them all the way.
- Never give up.

If you want to treat your bipolar disorder properly, you need to stop your substance use. To treat your substance abuse problem properly, you need to treat your bipolar disorder properly.

Identifying and Fighting Triggers

The **AAA Method**

AVOID Triggers When Possible

Don't Face Triggers **ALONE**

Distract Yourself by Getting
ACTIVE or Getting **AWAY**

Dealing with Depression without Abusing Substances

Characteristics of Depressive Thinking

Irrational Pessimism

Pessimism Feels "Realer" Than Real

Difficulty with Priorities

Coping with Depression

Helping Your Mood

Not Hurting Your Mood

Changing Your Thinking

Changing Your Behavior

Dealing with Family Members and Friends

Problems with Relationships

Hurt Feelings

Don't Count on Others for Your Recovery

Things May Get Worse before Getting Better

Follow-Through on Treatment

Explaining Can Help

Try to See Others' Point of View

Denial, Ambivalence, and Acceptance

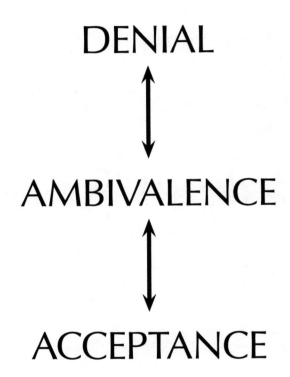

Reading Your Signals:
Recognizing Early Warning Signs of Trouble

READING YOUR SIGNALS

RECOGNIZING EARLY
WARNING SIGNS OF TROUBLE

MONITOR YOUR SYMPTOMS:
URGES TO USE ALCOHOL
AND DRUGS
MOOD PROBLEMS

BUILDING
UP TO
DRINKING AND DRUGGING

INDIVIDUAL PATTERNS

THE EARLIER, THE BETTER

MAKE CHANGES

Refusing Alcohol and Drugs:
Thinking It Through and Knowing What to Say

PRACTICING ALCOHOL AND DRUG REFUSAL

SNAPSHOT VERSUS VIDEO THINKING

BE PREPARED

DON'T LIE

DON'T BE DEFENSIVE

DON'T GIVE IN

REFUSE

Using Self-Help Groups

POSITIVE

_____

NEGATIVE

_____

THE PROGRAM

_____

THE FELLOWSHIP

_____

PROBLEM SOLVING

Taking Medication

BENEFITS

PROBLEMS

SOLVING THE PROBLEMS

SIDE EFFECTS

MOOD EFFECTS

ACCEPTANCE

TAKING MORE MEDICATION
THAN PRESCRIBED

Recovery versus Relapse Thinking: It Matters What You Do

"May as well" thinking
versus
"It matters what you do."

"It doesn't matter what I do."

"Who cares?"

"It does matter what I do."

Yes, it matters what you choose
to do:
Taking control of your life.

Hang up on your disease.

Taking Care of Yourself

Sleep

Regular Pattern

Avoid Caffeine

Exercise

Don't Toss and Turn

Talk to Your Treaters

Reducing HIV Risk

Follow Treatment Program

Avoid Risky Sex

HIV Testing

Don't Share Needles

Taking the Group with You

Summary of
Critical Ideas and Skills

STAY SOBER AND DRUG-FREE.

TAKE YOUR MEDICATION
AS PRESCRIBED.

DETECT DENIAL AND AMBIVALENCE.

TAKE CARE OF YOURSELF.

IDENTIFY AND FIGHT TRIGGERS.

RECOGNIZE EARLY WARNING SIGNS.

REMEMBER:
IT MATTERS WHAT YOU DO.

REVIEW SESSION HANDOUTS
TO REFRESH YOUR SKILLS.

Bulletin Board Material for All Group Sessions

INTEGRATED GROUP THERAPY FOR
FOR
BIPOLAR DISORDER
AND
SUBSTANCE ABUSE

CORE THEMES
FOR THIS GROUP

Central Recovery Rule

NO MATTER WHAT

- **DON'T DRINK**

- **DON'T USE DRUGS**

- **TAKE YOUR MEDICATION AS PRESCRIBED**

NO MATTER WHAT!

Routes to Recovery or Relapse

THOUGHTS ↔ BEHAVIORS ⟨→ RECOVERY
→ RELAPSE

Check-In

- Have you used any drugs or alcohol during the past week? If so, on how many days?

- How was your overall mood during the past week?

- Did you take your medication as prescribed during the past week? If not, why not?

- Did you face any high-risk situations or triggers for either substance use or mood problems in the past week? If yes, how did you deal with them?

⁅⁅⁅⁅⁅⁅⁅⁅⁅⁅⁅⁅⁅⁅⁅⁅⁅⁅⁅⁅⁅⁅⁅

Frequently Asked Questions
about Integrated Group Therapy

How does IGT integrate the treatment of bipolar disorder and substance use disorder?

There are several features that make IGT "integrated." First, a foundation of IGT is the concept that the same kinds of thoughts and behaviors that facilitate recovery from one disorder will facilitate recovery from the other disorder. Conversely, the same kinds of thoughts and behaviors that make recovery from one disorder more difficult will also make recovery from the other disorder more difficult. Thus, IGT focuses on "recovery thoughts" and "recovery behaviors" that facilitate recovery from both disorders. By the same token, IGT discusses "relapse thoughts" and "relapse behaviors" that can cause difficulties in the recovery from either disorder.

In addition to the focus on the *parallels* between the two disorders (as described earlier), IGT focuses on the *interaction* between the two disorders. In other words, IGT emphasizes the negative impact of substance use on the course of BD, and the negative impact of mood instability (frequently caused by BD medication nonadherence) on an SUD. Many people enter IGT because they are very concerned about *one* of their two disorders, but they may be much less worried about the other disorder. In fact, many patients who enter IGT groups are at best skeptical about the idea that they even *have* two disorders. For example, patients with severe BD may not see their SUD as particularly problematic, because they may not have experienced severe negative consequences of their substance use. However, they may be receptive to the idea that their substance use could make recovery from their BD more difficult.

Many people think of one of their disorders as *primary* (or, as some patients view it, "my *real* disorder"), and tend to minimize their other problem. IGT therefore asks patients to conceptualize themselves as having a *single disorder* (i.e., "bipolar substance abuse"). The treatment for bipolar substance abuse includes abstinence from drugs and alcohol, taking one's medication as prescribed, getting a good night's sleep, associating with the right people, and monitoring one's mood and the desire for drugs and alcohol. Each of these behaviors is designed to facilitate overall recovery in general, as opposed to recovery from one specific disorder.

Another way in which IGT is "integrated" is illustrated by the structure of the check-in that begins every group. The three cornerstones of the check-in are (1) substance use, (2) mood, and (3) medication adherence. All three issues are viewed as equally important. IGT is not a substance abuse group that happens to include people with BD. Nor is IGT a group for BD that happens also to talk about substance use. Both issues are seen as equally important, and the check-in at the beginning of each group demonstrates that concretely.

A final way in which IGT is integrated is illustrated by the group session topics. Whenever possible, IGT focuses on topics that are related to both disorders; an obvious example of this is Session 3, "Dealing with Depression without Abusing Substances." Another example is Session 5, "Denial, Ambivalence, and Acceptance," in which group members discuss these concepts in relation to both disorders.

Do you recommend having one leader or two leaders for IGT?

At McLean Hospital, we have always had one leader, and this has worked out quite well. However, much of our experience in running IGT has occurred in the context of a research study, in which a research assistant was always in the vicinity when a group was being conducted. This meant that if a clinical emergency arose during a session (e.g., a patient was intoxicated or manic), the patient experiencing a crisis could sit with the research assistant during the session and the clinician could meet with the patient individually after the session was completed. These emergencies happened very rarely, but they did occur; you should definitely develop a procedure to handle emergencies such as this when you run an IGT group. If you are working in a setting in which there will not be anyone else available to assist you in the case of such an emergency, then having a co-leader may be advisable. Thus, in summary, we have found a single leader to be perfectly adequate for IGT. However, emergency planning needs to considered when beginning an IGT group.

How many group members comprise an ideal size for IGT?

We have run IGT groups with as few as four patients and as many as 10. A group with fewer than four people generally does not allow for enough group interaction to be optimally helpful. Conversely, having more than 10 people in a group is also less than ideal; the check-in period takes up too much group time, and there is too little chance for people to discuss material related to the session topic when there are more than 10 people. An ideal size for an IGT group would be approximately six to eight patients.

When, if ever, would you tell someone to leave an IGT group permanently?

We have only rarely told someone to leave an IGT group permanently; this has occurred when someone in the group was threatening the recovery of other group members. Examples of behaviors that could lead to dismissal include offers to sell drugs to other group members, verbal or physical threats to either group members or the leader, or any behavior that undermines the purpose of the group. That said, we do not recommend that patients be dismissed from the group merely because they continue to use alcohol or drugs. One of the key goals of the group is obviously to help people stop their substance use. However, as long as they continue to try to use the group to facilitate their recovery, and as long as they do not interfere with the treatment of others, we do not believe that patients should be dismissed just because they continue to struggle.

Can the order of the group topics be switched?

Absolutely. Each group is self-contained, which means that it is not necessary to have attended previous groups to understand the content of a current group. The order of group topics listed in this book is merely a guideline and is not cast in stone.

Is it all right to mix people with bipolar I disorder and bipolar II disorder in an IGT group?

In our experience, approximately 80% of the people who have entered our IGT groups have had bipolar I disorder, but we have always also had people with bipolar II disorder. The key issue is that people entering the group should all believe (or at least should be willing to consider the idea strongly) that they, in fact, have BD. Having someone in the group who says, "I don't know what I'm doing here; I don't even have bipolar disorder," would be distracting and countertherapeutic for other group members. The issues related to the management of BD that are discussed in IGT are relevant to all subtypes of BD.

Would you mix drug users and people who use only alcohol in the same group?

Yes. Most of the people who have entered IGT have had both alcohol and drug use disorders, with nearly all having alcohol abuse or dependence. IGT does not distinguish between different drugs of abuse, but it encourages patients to abstain from both alcohol and drugs. Some patients who use more than one substance will be motivated to stop one substance and not another, but that situation commonly arises in all SUD treatment. We have experienced no difficulties over the years mixing those who primarily use drugs and those who use only alcohol. Rather, the commonality of having both an SUD and BD is much more important to IGT patients than differences in their preferred substance.

How long should an IGT group last?

In our studies, each IGT group session lasted an hour. However, we have visited a number of different programs in which IGT has been conducted, and the length of the session has varied. Some people have run IGT sessions for an hour, others for an hour and 15 minutes, and still others for an hour and a half. We know of one program that runs IGT sessions for 2 hours, with a 15-minute break in the middle. The first part of the session focuses on the check-in and the skill practice from the previous week, while the second part covers the session topic and the next week's skill practice. The length of the session may vary with the nature of the patient population and the size of the group; in general, we recommend more time for larger groups to allow for the greater number of check-ins and the increased interaction among group members.

Why do you ask in the check-in about the exact number of days of substance use during the previous week?

This is an important part of the check-in, because it helps build awareness of substance use and allows patients to track their progress. People who continue using drugs and alcohol when they know they shouldn't do so may not pay sufficient attention to their substance use behavior. It is common, for instance, for people who have just entered IGT to say, "I drank on 3 or 4 days last week." We suggest that group leaders follow up that type of statement with the question, "Was it 3 days or

4?" This is important, because a person who drank on 4 days last week and on 3 days this week has improved; conversely, drinking on 3 days last week and 4 days this week is evidence of backsliding. Drinking "3 or 4" days each week does not enable the therapist or the patient to know whether things are getting better or worse.

Would IGT work with people who have schizophrenia or schizoaffective disorder? What about people with major depressive disorder?

IGT has been adapted for use with patients who have either bipolar or psychotic disorders. This appears to have worked out quite successfully, in that the patients report finding the group helpful, group attendance is strong, and the leaders find the model appropriate for this population. Similarly, some programs have used IGT for patients with either BD or major depressive disorder, again with similar reports. Studies are currently being conducted to examine the efficacy of IGT in different patient populations. While these projects are going well, the final outcome data are not in yet.

Are there people whom you would exclude from entering an IGT group?

In general, IGT can be useful for a wide variety of patients, although their current state might make them inappropriate for attendance in a specific group. For example, someone who is hypomanic or manic would be disruptive in an IGT group, and should therefore not attend while in the middle of an acute episode. Moreover, people who are intoxicated can be disruptive in a group and cause others in the group to experience a great deal of craving and distress. We therefore typically recommended that people who have used drugs or alcohol on the day of the group not attend. While other group leaders may have somewhat different guidelines in this regard, we made that rule because asking people not to come to the group *intoxicated* would lead us to rely on a group member's own (often inaccurate) definition of what it means to be intoxicated.

People who absolutely deny having BD and/or a substance abuse problem are probably not good candidates for IGT either. One program, based in a mood disorder clinic that we visited, developed a clever solution to this issue by developing a "preparation" group for people with BD who denied having an SUD. This helped those patients to potentially reach a point at which they could benefit from IGT, by being willing at least to consider the idea that they might have these two problems.

What are the characteristics of a successful IGT group leader?

We have conducted IGT with a variety of types of group leaders. However, all had certain characteristics in common: experience leading groups and treating patients with SUDs. Whereas some leaders have had substantial experience and skill with CBT, others, without CBT experience, have had excellent results in IGT. Moreover, preexisting knowledge and experience with patients with BD can be helpful but has not been necessary as long as the group leader was willing to do some reading about BD and seek supervision from someone knowledgeable about that illness. Personal characteristics of a successful IGT leader are similar to the characteristics of good therapists in general: warmth, empathy, and good listening skills.

To what extent should the group leader comment on group process?

IGT does not focus on group process; rather, its foundations are based on cognitive-behavioral principles. That said, process is an inevitable component of any group. This becomes particularly clear when one examines the effect of the check-in on the rest of the group. When people report successful check-ins, the group session tends to go extremely well. When many group members have relapsed to substance use and are experiencing mood symptoms, the group session typically goes less well. If you find that the group process is interfering with the flow of the group, it may be worth commenting on that in a way that can move the group forward. If you are leading an IGT group and find that people are barely speaking after a difficult check-in, you might say something like "People seemed down after that check-in. I know that people can get discouraged, but it's a good thing that you are all here, ready to work on the issues we're going to discuss today. Maybe today's group can help people to turn the corner, so that the upcoming week will be a better week than this one."

Should IGT be run as an open group, in which patients can enter or leave at any time, or as a closed group, in which everyone enters together and finishes together?

We have run IGT in both ways, and either can be successful. In our first two studies, we conducted IGT as a closed group; in our third study, IGT was an open group. We currently run IGT in our clinical program as an open group, and that is what we recommend for most clinical programs. Running a closed group is logistically unwieldy, because you need to gather together a sufficient number of people all at once to comprise a viable group, and that can take some time. Moreover, if people leave the group, for whatever reason, then you are left with too few people to conduct a successful group. With an open group, the level of cohesiveness that can be achieved is not quite the same as in a closed group, but an open group is much more practical for a clinical program. Moreover, the infusion of new people throughout the course of the group can actually improve group dynamics by offering fresh perspectives on other people's issues.

Should people leave after completing 12 sessions of IGT, or can they stay in the group? If they stay beyond 12 weeks, how long do you recommend that they remain in the group?

In general, we recommend that people stay in IGT as long as they continue to find it helpful. In a clinical program, there is no reason for people to leave IGT after 12 weeks, unless they believe that they are no longer benefiting from the group. Some people may find that as topics are repeated, they benefit more from them the second time around. Other people have the opposite reaction, and say that they are bored after the first 12 weeks. The latter patients have probably achieved maximum benefit from IGT and should leave the group. As long as people continue to find IGT helpful, however, we recommend that they continue in the group.

References

American Psychiatric Association. (2000). *Diagnostic and Statistical manual of mental disorders* (4th ed., text rev.). Washington, DC: Author.

Babor, T. F., B. G. McRee, et al. (2007). Screening, Brief Intervention, and Referral to Treatment (SBIRT): Toward a public health approach to the management of substance abuse. *Subst Abuse* **28**(3): 7–30.

Bieling, P. J., R. E. McCabe, et al. (2006). *Cognitive-behavioral therapy in groups.* New York: Guilford Press.

Birmaher, B., D. Axelson, et al. (2009). Comparison of manic and depressive symptoms between children and adolescents with bipolar spectrum disorders. *Bipolar Disord* **11**(1): 52–62.

Brady, K., S. Casto, et al. (1991). Substance abuse in an inpatient psychiatric sample. *Am J Drug Alcohol Abuse* **17**(4): 389–397.

Brown, E. S., M. Garza, et al. (2008). A randomized, double-blind, placebo-controlled add-on trial of quetiapine in outpatients with bipolar disorder and alcohol use disorders. *J Clin Psychiatry* **69**(5): 701–705.

Brunette, M. F., & K. T. Mueser (2006). Psychosocial interventions for the long-term management of patients with severe mental illness and co-occurring substance use disorder. *J Clin Psychiatry* **67**(Suppl 7): 10–17.

Cassidy, F., E. P. Ahearn, et al. (2001). Substance abuse in bipolar disorder. *Bipolar Disord* **3**(4): 181–188.

Colom, F., E. Vieta, et al. (2003). A randomized trial on the efficacy of group psychoeducation in the prophylaxis of recurrences in bipolar patients whose disease is in remission. *Arch Gen Psychiatry* **60**(4): 402–407.

Craddock, N., M. C. O'Donovan, et al. (2005). The genetics of schizophrenia and bipolar disorder: Dissecting psychosis. *J Med Genet* **42**(3): 193–204.

Crits-Christoph, P., L. Siqueland, et al. (1999). Psychosocial treatments for cocaine dependence: National Institute on Drug Abuse Collaborative Cocaine Treatment Study. *Arch Gen Psychiatry* **56**(6): 493–502.

Dalton, E. J., T. D. Cate-Carter, et al. (2003). Suicide risk in bipolar patients: The role of comorbid substance use disorders. *Bipolar Disord* **5**(1): 58–61.

Drake, R. E., K. T. Mueser, et al. (1996). The course, treatment, and outcome of substance disorder in persons with severe mental illness. *Am J Orthopsychiatry* **66**(1): 42–51.

Dunn, C., L. Deroo, et al. (2001). The use of brief interventions adapted from motivational interviewing across behavioral domains: A systematic review. *Addiction* **96**(12): 1725–1742.

Dutra, L., G. Stathopoulou, et al. (2008). A meta-analytic review of psychosocial interventions for substance use disorders. *Am J Psychiatry* **165**(2): 179–187.

Edenberg, H. J., D. M. Dick, et al. (2004). Variations in GABRA2, encoding the alpha 2 subunit of the GABA(A) receptor, are associated with alcohol dependence and with brain oscillations. *Am J Hum Genet* **74**(4): 705–714.

Feltenstein, M. W., & R. E. See (2008). The neurocircuitry of addiction: An overview. *Br J Pharmacol* **154**(2): 261–274.

Ferri, M., L. Amato, et al. (2006). Alcoholics Anonymous and other 12-step programmes for alcohol dependence. *Cochrane Database Syst Rev* **3**: CD005032.

Frank, E., D. J. Kupfer, et al. (2005). Two-year outcomes for interpersonal and social rhythm therapy in individuals with bipolar I disorder. *Arch Gen Psychiatry* **62**(9): 996–1004.

Geddes, J. R., J. R. Calabrese, et al. (2009). Lamotrigine for treatment of bipolar depression: Independent meta-analysis and meta-regression of individual patient data from five randomised trials. *Br J Psychiatry* **194**(1): 4–9.

Goldberg, J. F., & M. Harrow (2004). Consistency of remission and outcome in bipolar and unipolar mood disorders: A 10-year prospective follow-up. *J Affect Disord* **81**(2): 123–131.

Goldstein, B. I., V. P. Velyvis, et al. (2006). The association between moderate alcohol use and illness severity in bipolar disorder: A preliminary report. *J Clin Psychiatry* **67**(1): 102–106.

Grant, B. F., F. S. Stinson, et al. (2004). Prevalence and co-occurrence of substance use disorders and independent mood and anxiety disorders: Results from the National Epidemiologic Survey on Alcohol and Related Conditions. *Arch Gen Psychiatry* **61**(8): 807–816.

Hasin, D. S., F. S. Stinson, et al. (2007). Prevalence, correlates, disability, and comorbidity of DSM-IV alcohol abuse and dependence in the United States: Results from the National Epidemiologic Survey on Alcohol and Related Conditions. *Arch Gen Psychiatry* **64**(7): 830–842.

Hawton, K., P. M. Salkovskis, et al. (1989). *Cognitive behavior therapy for psychiatric problems: A practical guide*. New York: Oxford University Press.

Hernandez-Avila, C. A., B. J. Rounsaville, et al. (2004). Opioid-, cannabis- and alcohol-dependent women show more rapid progression to substance abuse treatment. *Drug Alcohol Depend* **74**(3): 265–272.

Hettema, J., J. Steele, et al. (2005). Motivational interviewing. *Annu Rev Clin Psychol* **1**: 91–111.

Keck, P. E., Jr., S. L. McElroy, et al. (1997). Compliance with maintenance treatment in bipolar disorder. *Psychopharmacol Bull* **33**(1): 87–91.

Keck, P. E., Jr., S. L. McElroy, et al. (1998). 12-month outcome of patients with bipolar disorder following hospitalization for a manic or mixed episode. *Am J Psychiatry* **155**(5): 646–652.

Keller, M. B., P. W. Lavori, et al. (1986). Differential outcome of pure manic, mixed/cycling, and pure depressive episodes in patients with bipolar illness. *JAMA* **255**(22): 3138–3142.

Kendler, K. S., J. Myers, et al. (2007). Specificity of genetic and environmental risk factors for symptoms of cannabis, cocaine, alcohol, caffeine, and nicotine dependence. *Arch Gen Psychiatry* **64**(11): 1313–1320.

Kessler, R. C., R. M. Crum, et al. (1997). Lifetime co-occurrence of DSM-III-R alcohol abuse and dependence with other psychiatric disorders in the National Comorbidity Survey. *Arch Gen Psychiatry* **54**(4): 313–321.

Khantzian, E. J. (1985). The self-medication hypothesis of addictive disorders: Focus on heroin and cocaine dependence. *Am J Psychiatry* **142**(11): 1259–1264.

Kleber, H. D., R. D. Weiss, et al. (2007). [Work group on substance use disorders; American Psychiatric Association; Steering Committee on Practice Guidelines.] Treatment of patients with substance use disorders, second edition. *Am J Psychiatry* **164**(Suppl 4): 5–123.

Koob, G. F. (2009). Dynamics of neuronal circuits in addiction: Reward, antireward, and emotional memory. *Pharmacopsychiatry* **42**(Suppl 1): S32–S41.

Koob, G. F., & M. Le Moal (1997). Drug abuse: Hedonic homeostatic dysregulation. *Science* **278**(5335): 52–58.

Kranzler, H. R., & J. A. Tinsley, Eds. (2004). *Dual diagnosis and psychiatric treatment: Substance abuse and comorbid disorders*. New York: Marcel Dekker.

Lam, D. H., R. Burbeck, et al. (2009). Psychological therapies in bipolar disorder: The effect of illness history on relapse prevention—a systematic review. *Bipolar Disord* **11**(5): 474–482.

Lam, D. H., E. R. Watkins, et al. (2003). A randomized controlled study of cognitive therapy for relapse prevention for bipolar affective disorder: Outcome of the first year. *Arch Gen Psychiatry* **60**(2): 145–152.

Li, M. D., & M. Burmeister (2009). New insights into the genetics of addiction. *Nat Rev Genet* **10**(4): 225–231.

Madras, B. K., W. M. Compton, et al. (2009). Screening, brief interventions, referral to treatment (SBIRT) for illicit drug and alcohol use at multiple healthcare sites: Comparison at intake and 6 months later. *Drug Alcohol Depend* **99**(1–3): 280–295.

Miklowitz, D. J., M. W. Otto, et al. (2007). Psychosocial treatments for bipolar depression: A 1-year randomized trial from the Systematic Treatment Enhancement Program. *Arch Gen Psychiatry* **64**(4): 419–426.

Moss, H. B., C. M. Chen, et al. (2007). Subtypes of alcohol dependence in a nationally representative sample. *Drug Alcohol Depend* **91**(2–3): 149–158.

Mueser, K. T., A. S. Bellack, et al. (1992). Comorbidity of schizophrenia and substance abuse: implications for treatment. *J Consult Clin Psychol* **60**(6): 845–856.

Najavits, L. M. (2002). *Seeking Safety: A treatment manual for PTSD and substance abuse.* New York: Guilford Press.

Neves, F. S., L. F. Malloy-Diniz, et al. (2009). Suicidal behavior in bipolar disorder: What is the influence of psychiatric comorbidities? *J Clin Psychiatry* **70**(1): 13–18.

National Institute on Drug Abuse. (2009). *Comorbidity: Addiction and other mental illnesses* (NIH Pub. No. 08-5771). Washington, DC: Author.

Palmer, R. H., S. E. Young, et al. (2009). Developmental epidemiology of drug use and abuse in adolescence and young adulthood: Evidence of generalized risk. *Drug Alcohol Depend* **102**(1–3): 78–87.

Powers, M. B., E. Vedel, et al. (2008). Behavioral couples therapy (BCT) for alcohol and drug use disorders: A meta-analysis. *Clin Psychol Rev* **28**(6): 952–962.

Regier, D. A., M. E. Farmer, et al. (1990). Comorbidity of mental disorders with alcohol and other drug abuse: Results from the Epidemiologic Catchment Area (ECA) study. *JAMA* **264**(19): 2511–2518.

Salloum, I. M., J. R. Cornelius, et al. (2005). Efficacy of valproate maintenance in patients with bipolar disorder and alcoholism: A double-blind placebo-controlled study. *Arch Gen Psychiatry* **62**(1): 37–45.

Substance Abuse and Mental Health Services Administration. (2010). *Results from the 2009 National Survey on Drug Use and Health: National findings.* Rockville, MD: Author.

Tondo, L., B. Lepri, et al. (2007). Suicidal risks among 2826 Sardinian major affective disorder patients. *Acta Psychiatr Scand* **116**(6): 419–428.

U.S. Department of Health and Human Services. (1999). *Mental health: A report of the Surgeon General—executive summary.* Rockville, MD: Author.

Weiss, R. D. (2004). Treating patients with bipolar disorder and substance dependence: Lessons learned. *J Subst Abuse Treat* **27**(4): 307–312.

Weiss, R. D., M. L. Griffin, et al. (2000). Group therapy for patients with bipolar disorder and substance dependence: Results of a pilot study. *J Clin Psychiatry* **61**(5): 361–367.

Weiss, R. D., M. L. Griffin, et al. (2007). A randomized trial of integrated group therapy versus group drug counseling for patients with bipolar disorder and substance dependence. *Am J Psychiatry* **164**(1): 100–107.

Weiss, R. D., M. L. Griffin, et al. (2009). A "community-friendly" version of integrated group therapy for patients with bipolar disorder and substance dependence: A randomized controlled trial. *Drug Alcohol Depend* **104**(3): 212–219.

Weiss, R. D., W. B. Jaffee, et al. (2004). Group therapy for substance use disorders: What do we know? *Harv Rev Psychiatry* **12**(6): 339–350.

Weiss, R. D., M. E. Kolodziej, et al. (2000). Utilization of psychosocial treatments by patients diagnosed with bipolar disorder and substance dependence. *Am J Addict* **9**(4): 314–320.

Index